中华百草御膳

Chinese Hundreds of Herb-medicine
Imperial Cuisine
Prolonging Life

益寿篇

焦明耀　编著
Jiao Mingyao Editor

王涤寰　摄影
Wang Dihuan Photographer

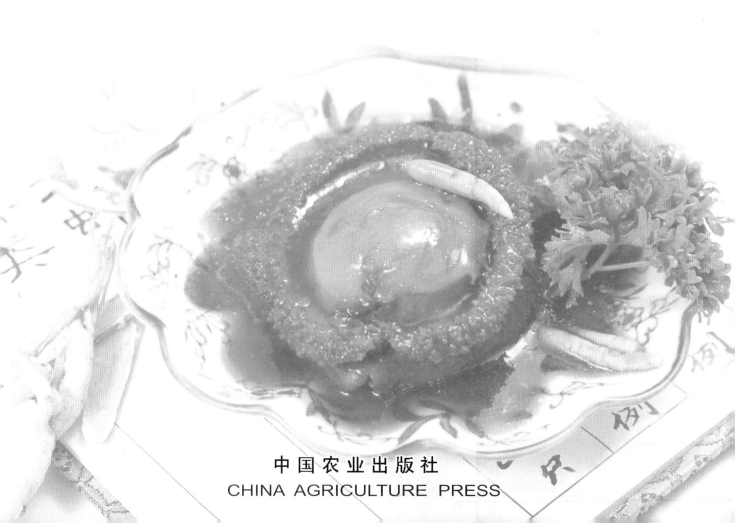

中国农业出版社
CHINA AGRICULTURE PRESS

作 者 简 介

　　焦明耀，曾任同仁堂御膳研究所常务副所长，同仁堂御膳餐饮有限公司总经理，兼任总厨，主要负责养生菜品的研制与开发。中国烹饪协会会员，中国药膳研究会会员，首都保健营养美食学会理事，东方美食学院客座教授。

　　多年来潜心研究养生御膳，理论与实际并重，古为今用，兼容并取，学名厨而不拘泥于成法，大胆创新而源于传统。在查阅了大量皇帝膳单的基础上虚心向烹饪大师学习请教，并结合传统"四季五补"理论与"现代养生"学说，辟出了一条以宫廷菜、官府菜及各地菜肴精华为基础的适合现代人们饮食特点的养生御膳之路。

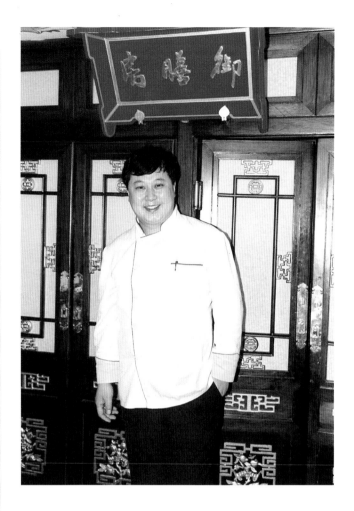

图书在版编目（CIP）数据

中华百草御膳．益寿篇／焦明耀编著；王涤寰摄．
北京：中国农业出版社，2001.10
ISBN 7-109-07233-9

Ⅰ.中...　Ⅱ.①焦...　②王...　Ⅲ.保健－菜谱－中
国　Ⅳ．TS972．161

中国版本图书馆 CIP 数据核字（2001）第 070048 号

出 版 人	沈镇昭
责任编辑	常一武　李　娜
出　　版	中国农业出版社
	（北京市朝阳区农展馆北路 2 号　100026）
发　　行	新华书店北京发行所
印　　刷	北京日邦印刷有限公司
开　　本	889mm × 1194mm　1/16
印　　张	7.25
字　　数	150 千
版　　次	2002 年 1 月第 1 版
	2002 年 1 月北京第 1 次印刷
印　　数	1～6 000 册
定　　价	43.50 元

（凡本版图书出现印刷、装订错误，请向出版社发行部调换）

Brief introduction of the author

　　Jiao Mingyao is an administrative assistant director of Tongrentang Imperial Cuisine Research Institute and he is General Manager and head cook of Tongrentang Imperial Cuisine Food Co., Ltd. He is in charge of research and development of dishes of nourishing life mainly. He is a member of China Cook Association, a member of China Herb-medicine Cuisine Association, a councilor of Capital Healthcare Nutriment & Cuisine Association and visiting professor of East Cuisine Academy.

　　He has researched nourishing imperial cuisine carefully for many years. He pays more attention to the theory and practice equally and learns from the ancient knowledge for the practice. He learns from the famous cook, but he never sticks to the accustomed rules and he is brave to create using the traditional culture. He learns from cook master modestly on the basis of consulting a great deal of the imperial cuisine and he has combined traditiona "Five tonifying of Four Seasons" with "Modern Nourishing" theory to develop the nourishing imperial cuisine road which is suitable for the modern people's diet characteristic on the basis of palace cuisine, authorities dishes and local cuisine essence.

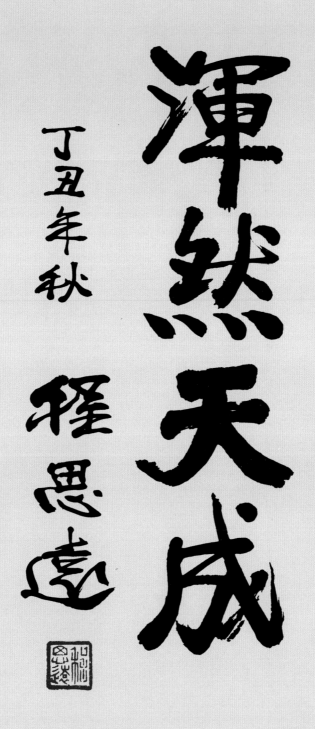

浑然天成

丁丑年秋 程思远

绪 论

21世纪，人们的饮食是以"健康合理"为主题。那么何为健康合理的饮食呢？健康合理的饮食是以人体在不同季节的不同生理状态为基础，采用适宜人体不同需求的食物，而饮食的进膳方法。早在《黄帝内经·素问·四气调神大论》中就有这样的记载："圣人春夏养阳，秋冬养阴，以从其根，故与万物沉浮于生长之门。逆其根则伐其本，坏其真矣"。这就是说，人们应顺应一年四季中的阴阳变化，在春季夏季要注意保养心肝，在秋季冬季要保养肺脾肾。所以，人们在饮食上也应该顺应这一养生之道的根本原则。要依照不同季节从饮食上适当的进行调补。

根据中国古老的"四季五补"理论认为："春季生补，夏季清补，秋季平补，冬季温补"。具体的说，春季人体肝火较旺，要食用具有健脾舒肝，有助于肝气生发作用的食物。夏季人体心火亢盛，外界的"暑湿"之邪当令，故此时要适时的食用具有清心祛暑，健脾利湿作用的食物。秋季空气干燥，"燥"邪当令，在饮食上应多食用具有滋阴润燥功效的食物。冬季人体的阳气潜藏，外界的气候寒冷，故此时人们应注意保养阳气。在饮食上要适当的食用一些具有温补脾肾，温通心阳作用的食物。

人们除了要注重食物的四季五补性，同时还要遑注重膳食的平衡。早在中国的古代，对于平衡膳食已有了粗浅认识，《黄帝内经》中说："毒药攻邪、五谷为养、五果为助、五畜为益、五菜为充、气味和而服之，以补精益气"。膳食平衡是指膳食中所供给的营养素与机体的生理需要保持平衡。其平衡膳食组成包括多种粮食类、肉类、蔬菜类、油脂类、水果类等。其基本要求是：1. 饮食要多样化，以保证营养素摄入的全面。其中要包括适量的肉类以提供机体生长发育和组织更新修复需要蛋白质。有富含丰富维生素的蔬菜和水果，以促进身体健康，增加免疫力。以及充足的无机盐以调节血浆电解质的平衡。在每天的饮食中还要包含一定量的谷类，以提供人体每天能量消耗所需的碳水化合物和脂肪。除此之外，每天还要摄入足够的膳食纤维，用以维持正常的排泄和预防一些疾病如心血管方面的疾病和某些消化系统的癌症。2. 各种营养素之间的比例要适当。如蛋白质、脂肪、碳水化合物三者之间要维持平衡，如果碳水化合物，脂肪的摄入不足就会影响蛋白质的合成。必须氨基酸的比例要适当。钙磷比值、锌铜比值、镁、钠、铁、碘等常量元素和微量元素应维持适宜的量。各种维生素的摄入也要全面，这样才能使其互相之间发挥协同作用。如维生素 A 只有和维生素 E 在一起才能发挥其抗氧化的作用……。

本书中所著菜谱中原料的选择，原料之间的互相搭配，是经过科学考究。原料的用量、也是通过科学的计算。菜肴的烹饪方法，都是经过多年的研究。可以满足人们对健康饮食的需求。但这只是对一般人群而定，一些特殊人群，还需在这些基础上，加以针对强化饮食。

倘若人类更注重科学养生膳食，那么人类的健康状况将得到极大的改善。

2001 年 12 月 26 日

Introduction

In twenty-first century,"the health and rational diet" is the main subject of the people's diet. What is health and rational diet?

The health and rational diet is a way of taking food,which the human body adopts the food benefiting the human body with different needs on the basis of different physiology of the human body in different seasons. There is recordation in 《Huangdi Neijing · Suwen · Siji Tiaoshen Dalun》:"Shengren Chunxia Yangyang,Qiudong Yangyin,Yicong Qigen,Gu Yu Wanwu Chenfu Yu Shengzhang Zhimen. Shuo Qigen Ze Faqiben, Huai Qi Zhenyi". That means the people shall be subject to the change of Yin and Yang of four seasons in a year. To protect and nourish the heart and liver in spring and summer. To protect and nourish the lung, spleen and kidney in autumn and winter. So,the people's diet shall be also subject to this basic principle of regimen and the people shall be nourished by the proper diet according to the different seasons.

The ancient "Five Nourishing in Four Seasons" theory of China thinks :"Chunji Shengbu, Xiaji Qingbu, Qiuji Pingbu, Dongji Wenbu". The meaning is that the people shall eat the food with function of tonifying the spleen, relaxing the liver and promoting the growth of liver qi because the liver fire of the human body is flourishing in spring. In summer, the heart fire of the human body is vigorous and the"hot weather wet" is prevailing, so the people shall eat the food properly with function of clearing the heart, eliminating the hot, tonifying the spleen and inducing diuresis. In autumn, the air is dry and the"dryness" is prevailing, so the people shall eat more food with function of nourishing yin and moistening the dryness. In winter, yang-qi is hid in the body and it is cold outside, so the people shall pay more attention to yang-qi and eat food properly with function of mild-nourishing of spleen and kidney and mild-penetrating of the heart-yang.

Except the people shall pay more attention to the five nourishing in four seasons nature of the food,the balance of the diet shall also be taken care. There was some knowledge about the balance of the diet in ancient time in China. 《Huangdi Neijing》 said:"Duyao Gongxie, Wugu

Weiyang,Wuguo Weizhu, Wuxu Weiyi,Wucai Weichong,Qiwei He Er Fuzhi, Yi Bujing Yiqi".
The diet balance means that it shall keep the balance between the nutriment and physiological need. The balance diet contains many kinds of food, meat, vegetables, fat and fruits, etc. The basic requirement is: 1. The diet shall be in diversification to guarantee the complete nutriment. Wherein, the proper quantity of the meat can provide the necessary protein for growth of organism and renewal of the tissue. The vegetables and fruits containing rich vitamins can promote the health of the body and enhance immunity. The sufficient inorganic salt can adjust the balance of electrolyte of blood plasma. In daily diet, some quantity of grains shall also be contained to provide the necessary carbohydrate and fat needed by the human body for energy of each day. Except this, the sufficient food fiber shall be ingested each day to keep the normal drainage and prevent some diseases and some cancer of digestive system. 2. The scale among the nutriment shall be proper. Such as protein , fat, carbohydrate shall be balance. If the carbohydrate and fat is insufficient, it will influence the composing of the protein. The scale of necessary amino acid shall be proper. The ratio of the calcium and phosphor, the ratio of copper and zinc, and the ordinary elements and micro elements, such as Mg, Na, iron and iodin shall be in proper quantity. The ingestion of each vitamin shall also be complete, only in this way, they can coordinate each other. For example, if put vitamin A and vitamin E together can resist oxidation, etc......

The selection of raw materials and arrangement of the raw materials in the menu written in the book is observed and studied by the science. The quantity of the raw materials used is also calculated scientifically. The cook way of the dishes has also been researched for many years. So all of these can satisfy the people's need for the health diet. But these are only suitable for the common people. For some specific people, the special food arrangement shall be paid more attention on this basis.

If the people pay more attention about the scientific regiment diet, then the people's health status shall be improved further.

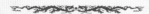

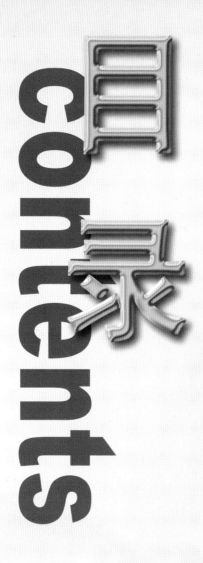

目录 contents

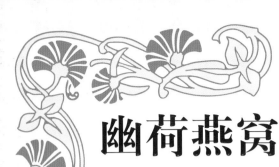

幽荷燕窝
Silent lotus and swallow nest

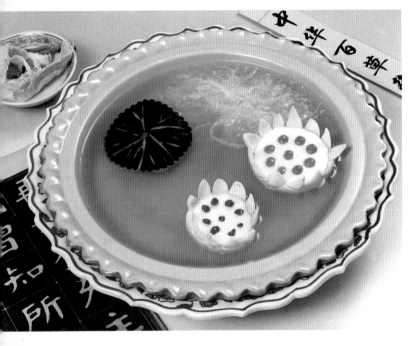

Main ingredient: 6g soaked swallow nest in the water.

Subsidiary ingredient: 2g lily, 10 green beans, 10 fruits of Chinese wolfberry, 50g Chinese watermelon, 25g culver breast, 1 egg white, 1 500g high-grade clear soup.

Flavouring: 3g iodin salt, 2g shellfish sauce.

Processing:

(1) Make the culver breast be fine and soft and then mix with egg white to make pastern. Inlay the fruit of Chinese wolfberry, green bean and lily into the pastern to make a lotus shape to be steamed for 4 minutes.

(2) Eliminate the impurity of the soaked swallow nest.

(3) Carve the tender Chinese lotus into lotus leaf shape and put them on the steamer to be steamed deeply.

(4) After seasoning the clear soup, put the swallow nest, lotus leaf and lotus flower in it.

Characteristic: The color is bright, the soup is clear and the shape is vivid.

主料：水发燕窝6克。

辅料：百合2克，青豆10粒，枸杞子10粒，冬瓜50克，斑鸠脯25克，蛋清1个，高级清汤1 500克。

调料：碘盐3克，瑶柱汁2克。

制作：

(1) 斑鸠脯打成茸与蛋清制成胶，分别镶入枸杞子、青豆、百合制成荷花上笼蒸4分钟。

(2) 水发燕窝去净杂质。

(3) 嫩冬瓜刻成荷叶，出水入味蒸透。

(4) 清汤调味后分别下入燕窝、"荷叶"、"荷花"。

特点：色泽明快，汤汁清澈，造型生动。

营养简析：

燕窝中含有丰富的多糖，斑鸠脯中有多量的"硒"元素，冬瓜、青豆中含有多量的维生素C。此菜具有健脾补肾、益寿抗衰老的功效。

发菜太极燕

Hair vegetable cooked with Taiji swallow

主料：水发燕窝 5 克，水发发菜 4 克。
辅料：咸蛋黄一个，高级清汤 50 克。
调料：碘盐 2 克，瑶柱汁 3 克。
制作：

(1) 水发燕窝去其杂质，发透。发菜温水涨发好后择净杂质加汤入味蒸 5 分钟。

(2) 咸鸭蛋黄蒸透切成两半。将发菜、燕窝分别放置深盘中缀以蛋黄使其呈太极状。

(3) 清汤入味勾二流芡浇入即可。

特点：黑白相间，口感清醇，回味绵厚。

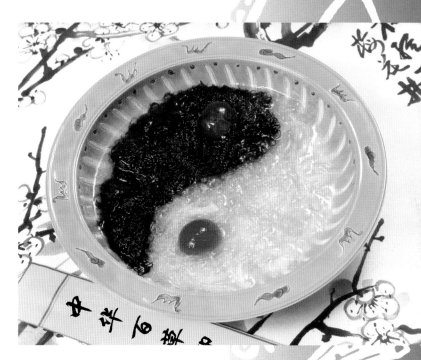

Main ingredient：5g soaked swallow in water，4g soaked hair vegetable．

Subsidiary ingredient：One salty egg yolk，50g high-grade clear soup．

Flavouring：2g iodin salt，3g shellfish sauce．

Processing：

(1) Eliminate the impurity of the soaked swallow nest and soak it deeply．After soaking the hair vegetable，eliminate the impurity and put it into the soup with flavouring to be steamed for 5 minutes．

(2) Cut the salty duck yolk into two pieces after it is steamed．Put the hair vegetable，swallow nest into a deep plate and put the egg yolk on it like Taiji shape．

(3) Season the clear soup and pour starchy sauce in it．

Characteristic：The color is black and white．The taste is light and pure with fragrant smell．

营养简析：

　　燕窝与发菜一起烹制具有补脾益肺，消瘿瘤的作用。发菜与燕窝中含有多种矿物质，而且种类全面。

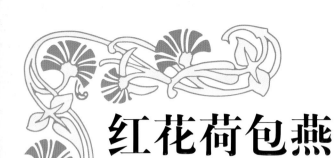

红花荷包燕
Saffron wrapping the swallow nest

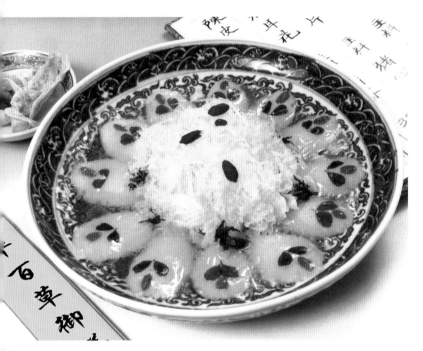

Main ingredient：10g soaked swallow nest.

Subsidiary ingredient：0.5g saffron, 2 tubes of Yuzi bean curd, one egg, 16 granules of fruit of Chinese wolfberry, a little bean seedling, 60g high-grade clear soup.

Flavouring：4g iodin salt, 3g shellfish sauce.

Processing：

(1) Eliminate the impurity after soaking the swallow nest and eliminate the water.

(2) Make the bean curd, egg, fruit of Chinese wolfberry and bean seedling together into pouch to be steamed for 4 minutes.

(3) Put the saffron into the clear soup to be steamed for 20 minutes to make saffron sauce.

(4) Put the bean curd around the swallow and pour starchy saffron sauce over the dish.

Characteristic：The color is splendid, the smell is fragrant and the taste is delicious.

主料：水发燕窝10克。

辅料：藏红花0.5克，玉子豆腐2管，鸡蛋1个，枸杞子16粒，豆苗少许，高级清汤60克。

调料：碘盐4克，瑶柱汁3克。

制作：

(1) 燕窝水发后漂净杂质，挤去水分。

(2) 玉子豆腐与鸡蛋、枸杞子、豆苗制成荷包，上笼蒸4分钟。

(3) 藏红花入清汤蒸20分钟，制成红花汁。

(4) 将玉子豆腐码在燕窝四周，红花汁入味后勾芡浇在菜肴上即可。

特点：色彩丰富，清远香醇，咸鲜适口。

营养简析：

　　燕窝与红花一同烹制具有补气活血养颜的功效。而且燕窝、玉子豆腐、鸡蛋中的氨基酸种类全面易于人体的吸收。

金凤戏燕窝

Golden phoenix playing with swallow nest

主料：斑鸠一只，水发燕窝4克。

辅料：鸽蛋10个，虫草1只，法香适量。

调料：老抽3克，碘盐1克，瑶柱汁2克。

制作：

 (1) 燕窝水发后处理干净，控净水分。

 (2) 净斑鸠出水后抹老抽炸至金黄色，入汤加入虫草、葱姜等同蒸40分钟至将脱骨。

 (3) 鸽蛋煮熟去皮炸成淡黄色，入味。

 (4) 将燕窝放置斑鸠四周撒入鸽蛋，扒以斑鸠原汁即可。

特点：色泽艳丽，香浓适中，形象生动。

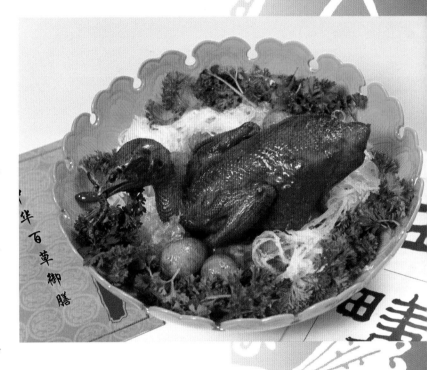

Main ingredient： One culver, 4g soaked swallow nest.

Subsidiary ingredient： 10 pigeon eggs, 1 Chinese caterpillar fungus, proper quantity of Faxiang plant.

Flavouring： 3g Laochou flavouring, 1g iodin salt, 2g shellfish sauce.

Processing：

(1) Clean the swallow nest after being soaked and eliminate the water.

(2) After boiling the clean culver lightly, roll in Laochou flavouring and deep—fry it into golden color. Put it in the soup, then put the Chinese caterpillar fungus shallot and ginger into the soup to be steamed for 40 minutes until the bone is boned.

(3) Peel the pigeon egg after boiling it and deep—fry it into golden color. Season it.

(4) Put the swallow around the culver and put the yolk on it. Pour the starchy culver sauce over the dish.

Characteristic： The color is flameboyant, the smell is fragrant and the shape is vivid.

营养简析：

  燕窝与斑鸠、冬虫夏草一起扒制具有补益肺脾肾、定喘的功效。而且斑鸠为高蛋白低脂肪的瘦肉型野禽，其肉质中所富含的"硒"元素具有抗癌、抗氧化的作用。

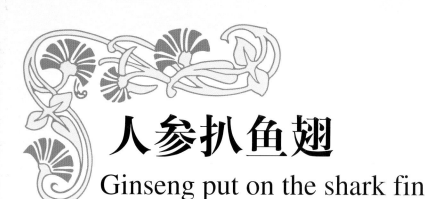

人参扒鱼翅
Ginseng put on the shark fin

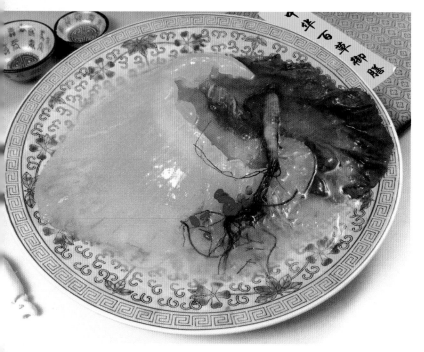

Main ingredient：One soaked shark fin.

Subsidiary ingredient：One mountain ginseng, a little fruit of Chinese wolfberry, 1 500g high—grade clear soup.

Flavouring：5g zinc salt, 3g ham sauce, 2g shellfish sauce, 6g tryptophan nutrition sauce.

Processing：

(1) Eliminate the fishy smell after boiling the shark fin lightly. Put the shark fin, mountain ginseng and fruit of Chinese wolfberry into the soup to be steamed until they are soft, then put them into the dish.

(2) After seasoning the sauce, pour over the shark fin.

Characteristic：The color is yellow and sleek, the taste is delicious with grand shape.

主料：水发鱼翅一块。

辅料：山参一只，枸杞子少许，高级清汤1 500克。

调料：锌盐5克，火腿汁3克，瑶柱汁2克，色氨酸营养液6克。

制作：

(1) 鱼翅出水后去掉腥味与山参、枸杞子同入高级清汤蒸至软烂拖入盘中。

(2) 原汁调味后扒在鱼翅上即可。

特点：色泽黄润，口感鲜浓，气势恢宏。

营养简析：

　　鱼翅与人参、枸杞子一同扒制具有补脾润肺，滋补肾精的作用。人参中含有多量的或类物质有强心的功效，对心衰有一定的治疗作用。

香菇鱼翅

Mushroom cooked with shark fin

主料：水发鱼翅一块。

辅料：香菇10个，香茅草少许，黄精0.1克，
　　　豆苗少许，高级清浓汤500克。

调料：蚝油10克，鲜菇老抽3克，木糖醇1克，
　　　色氨酸营养液6克。

制作：鱼翅洗净沙粒杂质，去掉腥味后加入
　　　黄精、香菇、香茅草同蒸至软烂。原汁
　　　调味收浓拖入盘中，撒豆苗即可。

特点：色泽红亮，菇香浓郁，口感软烂。

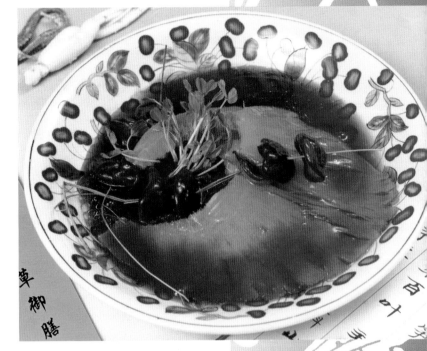

Main ingredient：One soaked shark fin.

Subsidiary ingredient：10 mushrooms, a little lemon-grass, 0.1g sealwort, a little bean seedling, 500g high grade clear soup.

Flavouring：10g oyster sauce, 3g fresh mushroom Laochou flavouring, 1g xylitol, 6g tryptophan nutrition sauce.

Processing：Eliminate the impurity of shark fin and peculiar smell. Put the sealwort, mushroom and lemon-grass together to be steamed until they are soft. Season the original sauce and make it be dense to put it in a plate and put some bean seedling on it.

Characteristic：The color is red and bright. The mushroom is fragrant and dense and the taste is soft.

营养简析：

　　鱼翅与香菇、黄精一同烹制具有补肾开胃，利肠道的功效。鱼翅中的鱼翅胶对血管硬化有一定的防治作用；香菇中含有多量膳食鲜味，可以减少人体对有害物质的吸收，还可降低血液中的胆固醇。

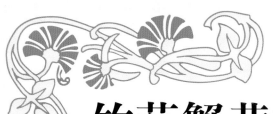

竹荪蟹黄翅

Zhusun cooked with the ovary and digestive glands of a crab and shark fin

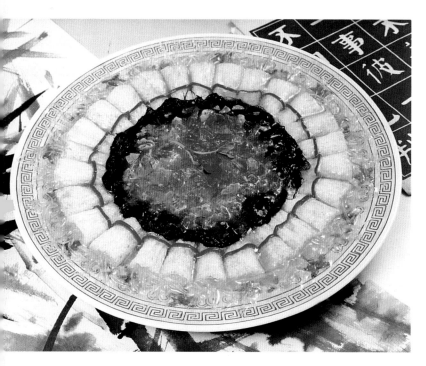

Main ingredient: 100g soaked shark fin.

Subsidiary ingredient: 2g dry Zhusun, 0.2g soaked hair vegetable, 50g ovary and digestive glands of a crab.

Flavouring: 5g zinc salt, 3g shellfish sauce, 1g sugar, 3g tryptophan nutrition sauce.

Processing:

(1) Soke the Zhusun in the cold water and cut it into one inch size.

(2) Put the soaked and seasoned shark fin into the Zhusun.

(3) Pour the hair vegetable and ovary and digestive glands of a crab in the middle of the dish.

Characteristic: The color is splendid, the taste is soft and fragrant.

主料：水发散鱼翅100克。

辅料：干竹荪2克，水发发菜0.2克，蟹黄50克。

调料：锌盐5克，瑶柱汁3克，糖1克，色氨酸营养液3克。

制作：

(1) 竹荪加入冷水发透，切成寸断。

(2) 将发好入味的鱼翅入竹荪中。

(3) 中间扒发菜、蟹黄即可。

特点：色彩丰富，口感软烂，鲜浓适口。

营养简析：

鱼翅与竹荪、蟹黄一同烩制具有补气强身的功效。其中，蟹黄中含有多种激素类物质，与富含多糖的竹荪在一起可以增强人体的抵抗力。

竹香黄金翅

Golden shark fin cooked with fragrant bamboo

主料：水发鱼翅 100 克。

辅料：高级浓汤 150 克，竹叶饭一碗 75 克。

调料：锌盐 3 克，火腿汁 1 克，瑶柱汁 2 克，
糖 1 克，色氨酸营养液 3 克。

制作：

(1) 鱼翅去净腥味，入浓汤蒸至软烂。

(2) 浓汁入味加鱼翅勾芡即可。

(3) 绿米加竹叶蒸熟。

特点：鱼翅色泽黄亮，竹叶饭碧绿清香，口
感香糯绵厚。

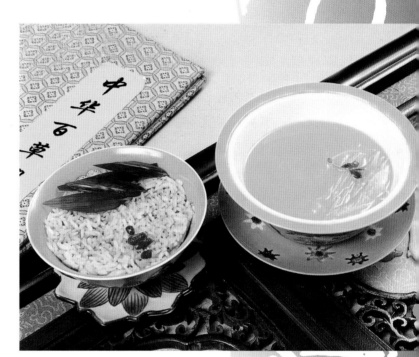

Main ingredient: 100g soaked shark fin.

Subsidiary ingredient: 150g high-grade dense soup,
75g one bowl of bamboo leaf rice.

Flavouring: 3g zinc salt, 1g ham sauce, 2g shellfish
sauce, 1g sugar, 3g tryptophan nutrition sauce.

Processing:

(1) Eliminate the fishy smell of the shark fin, put it
into the soup to be steamed until it is soft.

(2) Season the dense sauce and put the shark fin in
it with starch.

(3) Steam the green rice and bamboo leaf together.

Characteristic: The color of the shark fin is yellow
and bright. The bamboo leaf rice is green and fragrant
with delicious sticky rice taste.

营养简析：

　　鱼翅与竹叶饭一同食用
可以起到补脾润肺，清心利
尿的功效。并且，其中的色
氨酸营养液有助于将鱼翅中
的不完全蛋白质丰富为完全
蛋白质，易于人体的吸收。

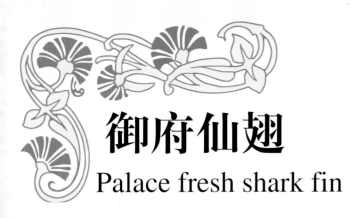

御府仙翅

Palace fresh shark fin

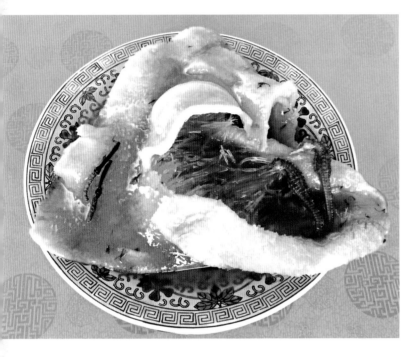

Main ingredient：One golden hook shark fin.

Subsidiary ingredient：1 000g high-grade dense soup, 1 fresh ginseng.

Flavouring：6g zinc salt, 4g shellfish sauce, 4g ham sauce, 6g chicken oil.

Processing：

(1) Soak the shark fin and eliminate the peculiar smell and impurity.

(2) Put the shark fin and ginseng into the dense sauce and put them to be steamed until they become soft.

(3) Pour them into the boiler and season them, then pour them over the shark fin.

Characteristic：The sauce is dense, fresh and fragrant. The color is yellow and sleek and the taste is soft and delicious.

主料：金勾翅一块。

辅料：高级浓汤1 000克，鲜人参1根，虫草二根，海马二根。

调料：锌盐6克，瑶柱汁4克，火腿汁4克，鸡油6克。

制作：

(1) 鱼翅水发，并去除异味及杂质。

(2) 鱼翅、人参入浓汁中，上笼蒸至软烂。

(3) 原汁倒入锅中，调好味，浇在鱼翅上即可。

特点：原汁鲜浓，绵厚，色泽黄润，口感软烂，鲜美无比。

营养简析：

鱼翅与人参一同蒸制具有补气润肺，健脾开胃的功效。鱼翅中含有丰富的鱼翅胶，粘多糖体，以及钙、铁、磷等多种营养素。人参中含有多种人参皂甙和氨基酸，可以提高人体心肌的射血能力。

太子鲍鱼
Taizi abalone

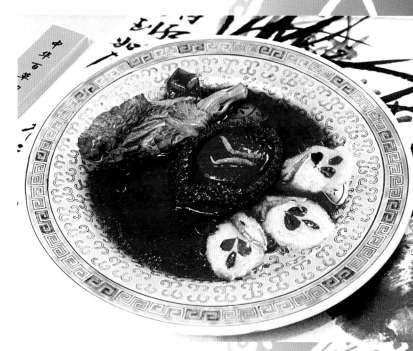

主料：网鲍一只。

辅料：太子参5只，芥兰1根，胡萝卜制成的
　　　玲珑球1个，豆腐荷包3个。

调料：美极酱油5克，鱼露3克，蚝油2克，
　　　冰糖1克。

制作：

(1) 干鲍鱼泡透后加太子参煲至劲道。

(2) 原汁加调料收至浓。

(3) 芥兰、玲珑球清炒，荷包摆在一侧
　　　即可。

特点：色泽红亮，香鲜浓郁，富有弹性。

Main ingredient：One abalone.

Subsidiary ingredient：5 Taizi ginseng, 1 leaf mustard,
1 exquisite ball made of carrot, 3 bean curd pouches.

Flavouring：5g Meiji soy sauce, 3g fish sauce, 2g
oyster sauce, 1g rock sugar.

Processing：

(1) After the dry abalone is soaked well, boil Taizi
ginseng and abalone together until it becomes
stretch.

(2) Put the flavouring in the original sauce and reduce
the sauce through simmering.

(3) Stir—fry leaf mustard and exquisite ball together
and put the pouches aside.

Characteristic：The color is red and bright and the
smell is fragrant with stretch.

营养简析：

　　鲍鱼与太子参、胡萝卜
一起烹制具有补脾益血的功
效。鲍鱼和豆腐中的氨基酸
的种类齐全易于人体合成蛋
白质。

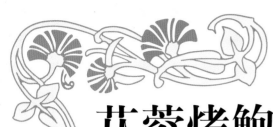

苁蓉烤鲍鱼
Roasted abalone with broomrape

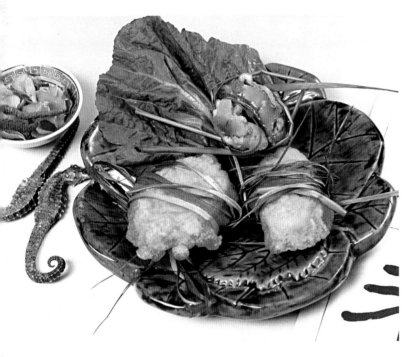

Main ingredient: 4 round granule abalone.

Subsidiary ingredient: 1g broomrape, proper egg paste, 2g lemon-grass.

Flavouring: 3g zinc saly, 2g brandy.

Processing:

(1) Mix the round granule abalone and broomrape powder and put them into the brandy.

(2) Stir the egg paste and roll the round granules in the paste.

(3) Roll in lemon-grass outside and put it into the oven to be roasted for 10 minutes.

Characteristic: The wine is fragrant, the surface is crisp and the inner is tender and aftertaste is long.

主料：圆粒鲍4只。

辅料：肉苁蓉1克，全蛋糊适量，香茅草2克。

调料：锌盐3克，白兰地2克。

制作：

(1) 圆粒鲍与肉苁蓉粉拌匀后入白兰地等。

(2) 全蛋糊和匀，包裹在圆粒鲍上。

(3) 将香茅草滚在外侧入烤箱烤10分钟即可。

特点：酒香浓郁，外酥里嫩，回味悠长。

营养简析：

　　鲍鱼与肉苁蓉一起烹制有补肾精，益肝血的功效。肉苁蓉中含有微量生物碱及结晶性、中性物质等，有降压、促进唾液分泌的作用。

明珠葵花鲍
Sunflower abalone with bright pearl

主料：圆粒鲍24粒。

辅料：金华火腿25克，香菇8只，桂圆16粒，
　　　高级清汤100克。

调料：锌盐5克，瑶柱汁4克。

制作：

(1) 圆粒鲍加入桂圆入清汤上笼蒸20
　　 分钟。

(2) 香菇发透去蒂。

(3) 火腿切成椭圆片。

(4) 将上述原料码成葵花形，加入清
　　 汤上笼蒸10分钟。

(5) 原汁调味勾芡浇上即可。

特点：形似葵花，刀工整齐，鲜香并重，口
　　　感爽滑。

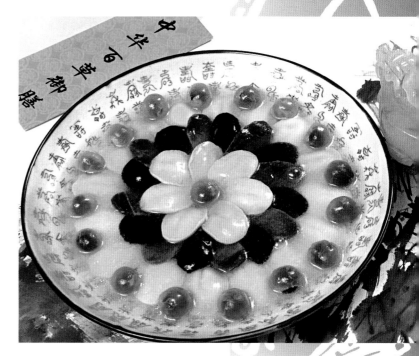

Main ingredient：24 round granules of abalone.

Subsidiary ingredient：25g Jinhua ham, 8 mushrooms,
16 granules of longan, 100g high—grade clear soup.

Flavouring：5g zinc salt, 4g shellfish sauce.

Processing：

(1) Put the round granules of abalone and longan
　　 into the soup to be steamed for 20 minutes.

(2) Soak the mushrooms and cut out the pedicels.

(3) Cut the ham into ellipse pieces.

(4) Put the above ingredients together like sunflower
　　 shape and put the clear soup into them, then
　　 steam them for 10 minutes.

(5) Pour the starchy original sauce over them.

Characteristic：The cut is in order, the dish is fragrant
and fresh with well feel.

营养简析：

　　圆粒鲍与桂圆一同蒸制
具有滋补肝血，养心安神的
功效。鲍鱼中所缺的氨基酸
可被香菇中的必须氨基酸所
补充，有利于人体的吸收。

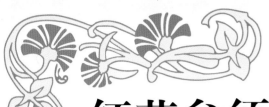

红花参须鲍

Abalone cooked with saffron and ginseng fiber

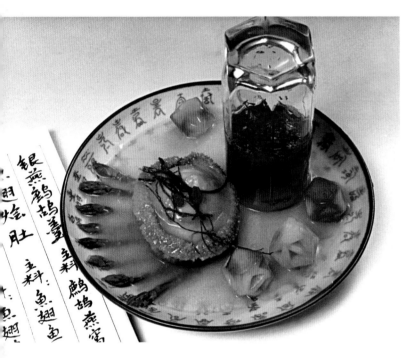

Main ingredient: One fresh abalone with black and blue border.

Subsidiary ingredient: 0.5g saffron, 1.5g ginseng fiber, 8 fresh bamboo shoots, 3 carrot balls, 1 blue bamboo ball, 50g high-grade clear soup.

Flavouring: 5g zinc salt, 4g shellfish sauce.

Processing:

(1) Blue border abalone, saffron and ginseng fiber are cooked to reduce sauce, then put them into a plate.

(2) Steam the saffron in the soup, season it and put it into a glass. Reverse the glass in one side of the plate.

(3) Stir-fry the carrot, blue bamboo shoot balls and asparagus together.

Characteristic: The taste is fresh and delicious. And using the saffron as vegetable is a special way.

主料：鲜青边鲍一只。

辅料：藏红花0.5克，人参须1.5克，鲜芦笋尖8根，
　　　胡萝卜球3个，青笋球1个，高级清汤50克。

调料：锌盐5克，瑶柱汁4克。

制作：

(1) 青边鲍与藏红花、参须煲制后收汁入盘。

(2) 红花入汤蒸后调味盛入杯中，倒扣在盘中一侧。

(3) 胡萝卜球、青笋球、芦笋尖清炒。

特点：口味鲜浓，以花入菜，别具一格。

营养简析：

　　鲍鱼与藏红花、人参一同烹制具有补气，活血补血的作用。其中的笋类与胡萝卜中含有多量的维生素A，以及多糖类物质，可起到抗衰老的功效。

杞红鲍鱼

Red abalone cooked with fine and soft astraglus base

主料：圆粒鲍9只。

辅料：杞茸汁100克，西洋参0.5克，高级清汤150克。

调料：锌盐5克，鲜味汁6克。

制作：

    （1）鲍鱼出水后与杞茸汁、西洋参同煲两小时。

    （2）清汤入味勾芡入鲍鱼即可。

特点：汤汁清澈，鲍鱼红润，鲜咸利口。

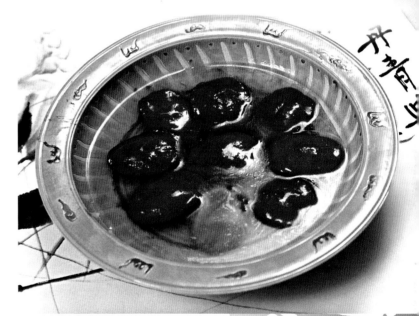

Main ingredient：9 round granules of abalone.

Subsidiary ingredient：100g fine and soft astraglus base, 0.5g ginseng, 150g high—grade clear soup.

Flavouring：5g zinc salt, 6g fresh sauce.

Processing：

(1) After boiling the abalone a little, boil the fine and soft astraglus base and ginseng together for 2 hours.

(2) Season the clear soup and pour the starchy sauce over the abalone.

characteristic：The soup is clear, the zbzlone is ruddy and the dish is salty and dainty with fragrance.

营养简析：

    鲍鱼与枸杞子、西洋参一同烧制具有滋阴补血的功效。西洋参中含有10多种人参皂甙、糖类、氨基酸，有促进肾上腺皮质激素分泌的作用，能增强人体的免疫力。

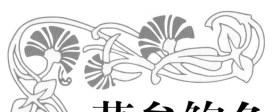

芪参鲍鱼

Abalone cooked with ginseng and astraglus base

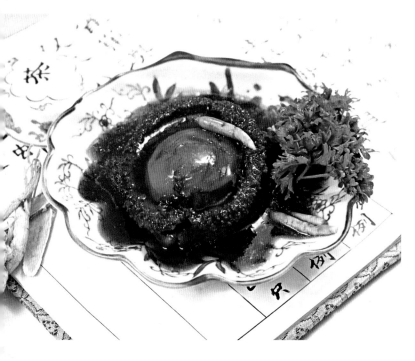

Main ingredient：One fresh abalone with blue border.

Subsidiary ingredient：3g astraglus base, 2g Taizi ginseng, 1g saffron, 1 000g high-grade clear soup.

Flavouring：25g fermented soya beans oil, 25g fresh sauce, 15g saffron sauce, 10g rock sugar.

Processing：

(1) Clean the fresh abalone with blue border.

(2) Cook the astraglus base and Taizi ginseng together for 12 hours.

(3) Color it, season it and reduce the sauce by stir-frying.

Characteristic：The color is red with moisture. The taste is fresh and delicious. The nutrition is rich.

主料：鲜青边鲍鱼1只。

辅料：黄芪3克，太子参2克，藏红花1克，高级清汤1 000克。

调料：豉油25克，鲜味汁25克，红花汁15克，冰糖10克。

制作：

(1) 鲜青边鲍初步处理干净。

(2) 与黄芪、太子参等同煲12小时左右。

(3) 收汁调色调味即可。

特点：色泽红润，口味鲜美，营养丰富多样。

营养简析：

　　鲍鱼与黄芪、太子参、藏红花一同烹制具有补气活血，抗衰老的作用。鲍鱼中含有丰富的蛋白质、烟酸、多不饱和脂肪酸、多种无机盐等成分。

银雀雏凤

Silver bird played with young phoenix

主料：干贝茸25克。

辅料：鸽蛋8个，西兰花100克，鸡茸50克，
藏红花0.1克，黄精0.2克，细粉丝30
克，高级清汤25克。

调料：锌盐4克，鸡油2克。

制作：

(1) 将干贝茸与鸡茸制成凤身。

(2) 鸽蛋制成头，黄精蒸透打碎制成
凤冠，与凤身合成雏凤上笼蒸6分
钟，扒以浓汁。

(3) 细粉丝炸后撒上红花。

(4) 西兰花清炒分入盘中即可。

特点：造型逼真，鲜浓爽口，回味无穷。

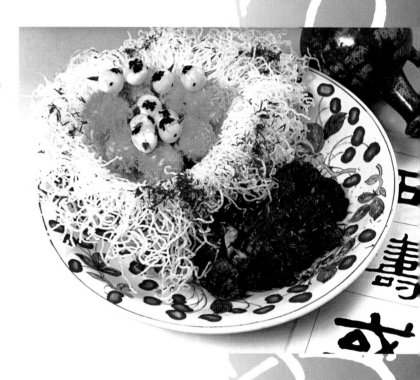

Main ingredient: 25g fine and soft dried scallop.

Subsidiary ingredient: Eight pigeon's eggs, 100g
green cauliflower, 50g fine and soft chicken, 0.1g
saffron, 0.2g sealwort, 30g thin vermicelli, 25g high-
grade clear soup.

Flavouring: 4g zinc salt, 2g chicken oil.

Processing:

(1) Make fine and soft dried scallop, soft and fine
chicken into the body of a phoenix.

(2) Make the pigeon's eggs be the phoenix's head,
steam the sealwort and mince it to be the
phoenix's crest. Steam the young phoenix for
six minutes and pour the sauce over the dish.

(3) After the thin vermicelli is deep-fried, pour the
saffron over the dish.

(4) Stir-fry the green cauliflower and put the dish
on a plate.

Characteristic: The shape is vivid and it tastes
absolutely delicious.

营养简析：

　　干贝与藏红花、黄精一
同扒制具有补肾滋阴潜阳的
功效。其中的鸽蛋、鸡茸与干
贝中的氨基酸种类齐全易于
人体的吸收。

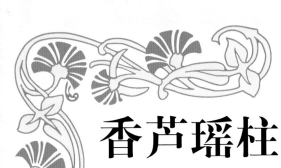

香芦瑶柱
Spicy aloe cooked with shellfish

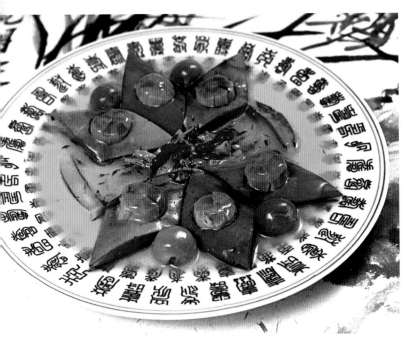

Main ingredient: 8 dried scallops.

Subsidiary ingredient: 6 pieces of aloes, 4 longan, a little fruit of Chinese wolf—berry, 75g high—grade soup.

Flavouring: 4g zinc salt, 2g shellfish sauce.

Processing:

(1) Brew the soaked shellfish into the aloe and steam it for four minutes.

(2) Peel the fresh longan into the soup and put shellfish's shreds, the fruit of Chinese wolf—berry over the dish.

Characteristic: It is decorated with red fruit of Chinese wolf—berry between green and yellow. The shape is vivid, colourful and lustrous. It tastes fresh and salty.

主料：干贝8粒。

辅料：芦荟6块，桂圆4只，枸杞子少许，上汤75克。

调料：锌盐4克，瑶柱汁2克。

制作：

(1) 水发瑶柱酿入芦荟中入笼蒸4分钟。

(2) 鲜桂圆去皮入汤与瑶柱丝、枸杞子同扒其上即可。

特点：黄绿相间缀以杞红，色泽明快，口味鲜咸。

营养简析：

　　干贝与芦荟、桂圆、枸杞子一同烹制具有滋补心肾、清肝火、通便的功效。其中芦荟含有丰富的粘性物质可有效的保留人体内的水分，有美容的功效。

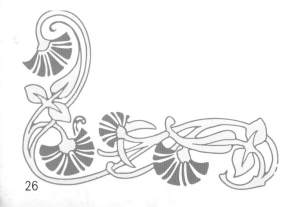

红参瑶柱

Red ginseng shellfish

主料：水发干贝8粒。

辅料：红参0.5克，冬瓜环4只，斑鸠茸25克，
　　　高级清汤3两。

调料：锌盐0.5克，瑶柱汁4克。

制作：

（1）四只水发干贝酿入处理好的冬瓜
环中。

（2）另两只干贝搓成丝与斑鸠脯茸制
成球。

（3）上述两种原料与红参及高级清汤
共同蒸10分钟。

（4）原汁调味倒回即可。

特点：汤鲜味美，色泽和谐，口感清醇。

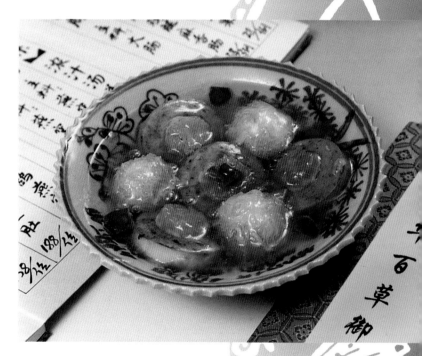

Main ingredient：8 soaked dried scallops.

Subsidiary ingredient：0.5g ginseng, 4 wax gourd
circles, 25g soft and fine culver, 3 taels high—grade
clear soup.

Flavouring：0.5 zinc salt, 4g shellfish's sauce.

Processing：

(1) Brew four soaked dried scallops into the worked
wax gourd circles.

(2) Make the other dried scallops shreds and soft
and fine culver be a ball.

(3) Steam the above ingredients, red ginseng and
high—grade clear soup together for ten minutes.

(4) Season the original sauce and pour it back.

Characteristic：The soup is fresh, fragrant and delicious
with harmonious colour and lustre.

营养简析：

　　瑶柱与红参、冬瓜一同
蒸制使其具有补肾利尿的功
效。干贝与斑鸠中的氨基酸
种类齐全易于人体的吸收。

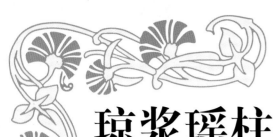

琼浆瑶柱
Shellfish with fine and delicious wine

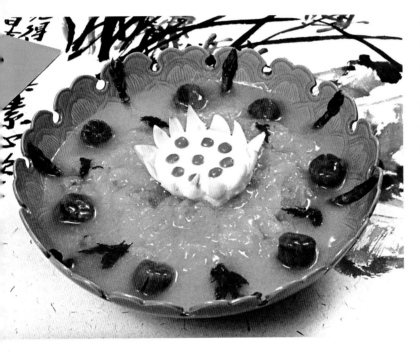

Main ingredient: 8 dry shellfishes.

Subsidiary ingredient: 150g dry fish tripe, 25g fine and soft culver, 9 green beans, 0.1g saffron, 1 fresh lily, 150g high—grade dense soup.

Flavouring: 7g zinc salt, 8g shellfish ham sauce, 3g chicken oil, 2g sugar.

Processing:

(1) Make lotus with fresh lily, fine and soft culver breast and green beans and steam them for 4 minutes.

(2) After cleaning the dry shellfish and eliminating the tendons, steam it with saffron and fish tripe together for 35 minutes.

(3) Take out the original sauce and season it, the pour the starchy sauce over it. Boil the oil with ingredients.

Characteristic: The sauce is dense and delicious and fragrant competing the fine and delicious wine.

主料：干瑶柱8只。

辅料：油发鱼肚150克，斑鸠茸25克，青豆9粒，藏红花0.1克，鲜百合1个，高级浓汤150克。

调料：锌盐7克，瑶柱火腿汁8克，鸡油3克，糖2克。

制作：

(1) 鲜百合与斑鸠脯茸、青豆等制成莲花，上笼蒸4分钟。

(2) 干贝洗净去筋后与藏红花、鱼肚同蒸35分钟。

(3) 原汁滗出调味勾芡，明油加入原料烧开即可。

特点：汁浓味美，绵软醇厚，赛比琼浆。

营养简析：

瑶柱与藏红花、鲜百合一同烧制具有滋补心肾，活血舒肝的功效。其中鱼肚、斑鸠、青豆中含有粘蛋白、氨基酸、维生素C等多种营养素。

八珍鱼肚

Eight precious ingredients with fish tripe

主料：油发鱼肚75克。

辅料：斑鸠苴50克，大虾粒10克，淮山粒10克，草菇粒10克，牡蛎粒10克，枸杞子10克，肉苁蓉1克，鲍鱼粒5克，高级清汤50克。

调料：锌盐6克，瑶柱火腿汁8克，鸡油3克。

制作：

(1)"八珍原料"拌匀入味。

(2)油发鱼肚控干水分，抹上八珍料，上笼蒸6分钟扒汁即可。

特点：造型整齐，选料丰富，口味咸鲜，口感松软。

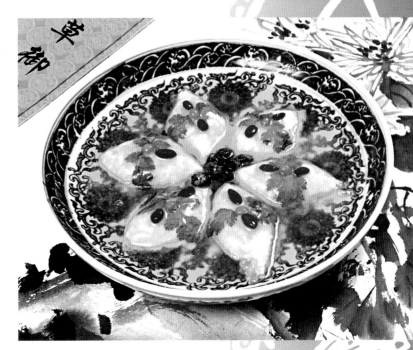

Main ingredient：75g dry fish tripe.

Subsidiary ingredient：50g fine and soft culver, 10g big shrimp granules, 10g Huaishan yam granules, 10g straw mushroom granules, 10g syster granules, 10g fruit of Chinese wolfberry, 1g broomrape, 5g abalone granules, 50g high—grade clear soup.

Flavouring：6g zinc salt, 8g shellfish ham sauce, 3g chicken oil.

Processing：

(1) Mix the "Eight precious ingredients" and season them.

(2) Clear the damp of dried fish tripe, roll in eight precious ingredients and steam them for 6 minutes. At last, pour the starchy sauce over them.

Characteristic：The shape is in order, the ingredients are rich, the taste is salty and fresh and the taste is soft and short.

营养简析：

　　鱼肚与山药、枸杞子、肉苁蓉及八珍原料一同烹制具有大补五脏精气的功效。而且，其中的营养成分全面。

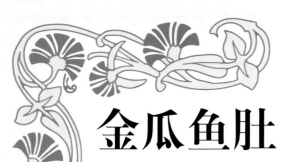

金瓜鱼肚

Fish tripe cooked with golden melon

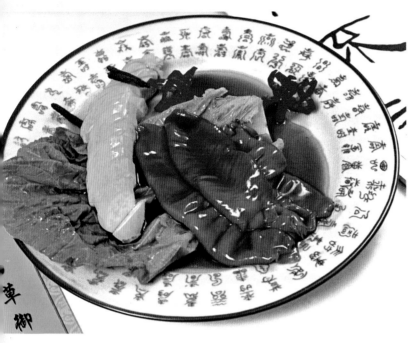

Main ingredient: 3 soaked eel tripes.

Subsidiary ingredient: 1 small golden melon, 2 piper longums, 100g fruit of Chinese wolfberry.

Flavouring: 4g zinc salt, 6g fresh sauce, 1g sugar.

Processing:

(1) After the fruit of Chinese wolfberry is soaked in the water, make it be fine and soft.

(2) Boil the soaked fish tripes, piper longums and fine and soft fruit of Chinese wolfberry together for 40 minutes and use the original sauce to season.

(3) After the small golden melon is stir-fried, put it into a plate and pour the sauce over it.

Characteristic: The color of the tripe is red and bright, the taste is sticky rice fragrant, the golden melon is orange and the taste is crisp.

主料：水发鳗鱼肚3根。

辅料：小金瓜1个，毕菝2根，枸杞子100克。

调料：锌盐4克，鲜味汁6克，糖1克。

制作：

(1) 杞子水发后打成碎茸。

(2) 水发鱼肚、毕菝入枸杞子茸中煲40分钟原汁调味。

(3) 小金瓜清炒后分入盘中，扒汁。

特点：鱼肚色泽红亮，口感香糯，金瓜橘黄，口感爽脆。

营养简析：

　　鱼肚与毕菝、枸杞子一同烹制具有温补脾肾的功效。小金瓜中含有丰富的维生素E可起到排除体内自由基、抗衰老的作用。

玉珠鱼肚
Pearl with fish tripe

主料：水发鳗鱼肚两根。

辅料：黄精0.2克，桂圆8粒，西兰花100克，
　　　高级清汤100克。

调料：锌盐4克，鲜味汁4克。

制作：

　　(1) 西兰花与桂圆清炒后垫在盘中。

　　(2) 水发鱼肚与黄精同蒸20分钟后原
　　　　汁入味扒在菜品上即可。

特点：红绿相间，色泽明快，口味鲜浓，口感
　　　软糯。

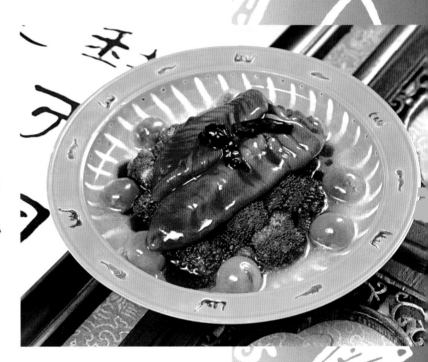

Main ingredient： Two soaked eel tripes.

Subsidiary ingredient： 0.2g sealwort, 8 granules of longan, 100g green cauliflower, 100g high—grade clear soup.

Flavouring： 4 zinc salt, 4g fresh sauce.

Processing：

(1) After the green cauliflower and longan are stir—fried, put them into a plate.

(2) Steam the soaked fish tripe and sealwort together for 20 minutes and pour the original sauce over the dish.

Characteristic： The color is red, green and bright. The taste is fresh and fragrant with sticky rice smell.

营养简析：

　　鱼肚与黄精、桂圆一同
扒制具有补肾健脾，养心血
的功效。

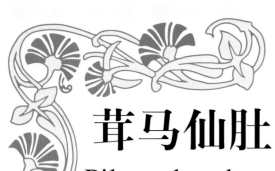

茸马仙肚

Pilose deer horn, sea horse and celestial tripe

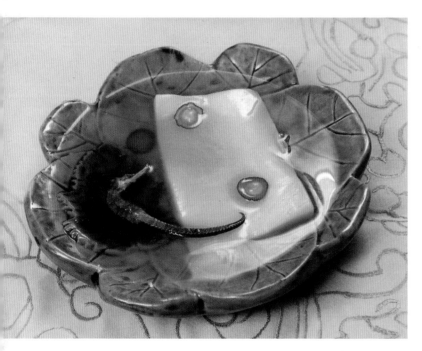

Main ingredient: 80g soaked fish tripe, 100g high-grade clear soup.

Subsidiary ingredient: 1 sea horse, 3 pilose deer horns.

Flavouring: 3g zince salt, 6g fresh sauce.

Processing:

(1) Steam the soaked fish tripe, sea horse and pilose deer horn together in the soup for 20 minutes.

(2) Take out the original soup and season it.

Characteristic: The taste is original and the sauce is dense and fragrant.

主料：水发鱼肚80克、高级清汤100克。

辅料：海马1只，鹿茸3片。

调料：锌盐3克、鲜味汁6克。

制作：

(1) 将水发鱼肚与经过初步处理的海马、鹿茸同入汤中同蒸20分钟。

(2) 原汁倒出调味即可。

特点：原汁原味，汁浓味厚。

营养简析：

鱼肚与海马、鹿茸一同烹制具有健脾益气、温补肾阳、以后天养先天的作用。

神仙鱼肚
Celestial fish tripe

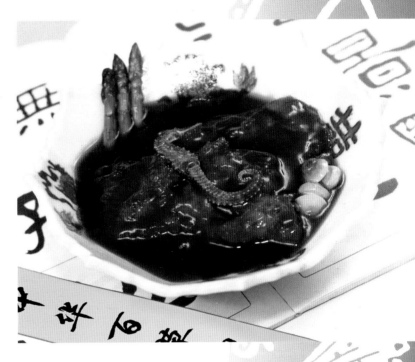

主料：油发广肚150克。

辅料：黄精0.1克，海马1只，草菇心3粒，鲜
　　　芦笋尖3根，高级清汤。

调料：老抽3克，蚝油2克，鱼露1克，糖0.5克。

制作：(1) 鱼肚处理好后入黄精、海马、草菇
　　　　　等同蒸至软烂。

　　　(2) 原汁入锅调味调色。

　　　(3) 鲜芦笋清炒垫入盘中即可。

特点：色泽红润，胶质丰富，口感滑糯，食之
　　　赛仙。

Main ingredient：150g Guangdu tripe soaked.

Subsidiary ingredient：0.1g sealwort, 1 sea horse, 3 granules of straw mushroom, 3 fresh bamboo shoots, high-grade clear soup.

Flavouring：3g LaoChou Flavouring, 2g oyster sauce, 1g fish oil, 0.5g sugar.

Processing：

(1) After treating the fish tripe, seam it with sealwort, seahorse and straw mushroom together until they become soft.

(2) Put the original sauce into the boiler to be seasoned and colored.

(3) Stir-fry the fresh bamboo shoots and put them on the bottom of the plate.

Characteristic：The color is red with moisture, the colloid is rich, the taste is delicious with sticky rice smell competing the celestial being.

营养简析：

　　鱼肚与富含多糖类物质的草菇、芦笋一同烹制可起到延缓细胞衰老的作用。其中加入海马、黄精后还可起到补肾阳、益脾气的作用。

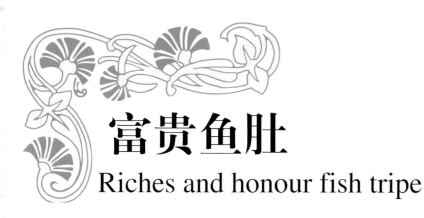

富贵鱼肚

Riches and honour fish tripe

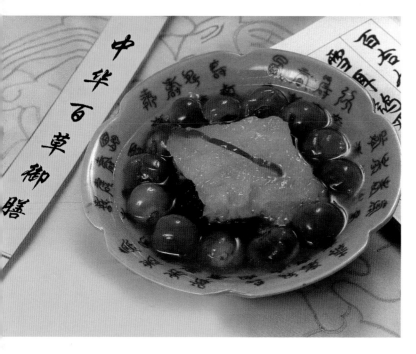

Main ingredient: 35g deep-fried fish tripe.

Subsidiary ingredient: 13 granules of fresh longan, 0.1g cornel, 150g high-grade clear soup.

Flavouring: 2g zinc salt, 2g ham sauce, 2g chicken oil.

Processing:

(1) Steam the cornel and longan together with the soup for 10 minutes.

(2) After the fish tripe is boiled lightly, put it into the cornel and longan sauce and season it.

Characteristic: The color is bright, the taste is fresh and sweet.

主料：油发鱼肚 35 克。

辅料：鲜桂圆 13 粒，山萸肉 0.1 克，高级清汤 150 克。

调料：锌盐 2 克，火腿汁 2 克，鸡油 2 克。

制作：

(1) 山萸肉与桂圆入清汤蒸 10 分钟。

(2) 鱼肚出水后加入山萸桂圆汁调味即可。

特点：色泽明快，咸鲜适中，回味微甜。

营养简析：

鱼肚与山萸肉、桂圆一同烹制可起到健脾养心，收敛肾精的作用。

鸳鸯红花肚

Mandarin duck and saffron tripe

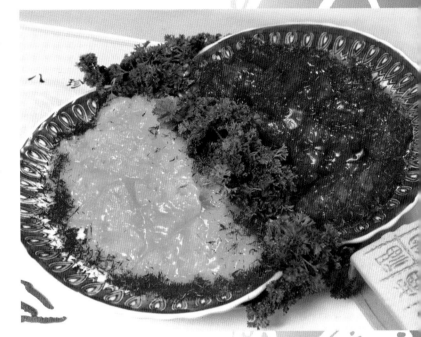

主料：油发广肚 500 克。

辅料：藏红花 0.2 克，黄精 0.2 克，高级浓汤
　　　150 克。

调料：锌盐 6 克，糖 4 克，鲜味汁 4 克，红油
　　　12 克，鸡油 8 克。

制作：

　　　(1) 一半鱼肚与藏红花浓汁同黄精烧。

　　　(2) 另一半鱼肚与黄精一起干烧。

特点：红黄相应，口味丰富，口感滑软。

Main ingredient：500g pan—fried Guang Du tripe.

Subsidiary ingredient：0.2g saffron, 0.2g sealwort,
150g high—grade dense soup.

Flavouring：6g zinc salt, 4g suger, 4g fresh sauce,
12g pepper oil, 8g chicken oil.

Processing：

(1) Braise one half fish maw, saffron and sealwort
　　together in dense sauce.

(2) Braise the other half fish maw with sealwort in
　　soy sauce.

Characteristic：The colour is red and green. It is soft,
sleek and delicious.

营养简析：

　　鱼肚与红花、黄精一同
烹制具有补脾益肾，活血舒
肝的功效。

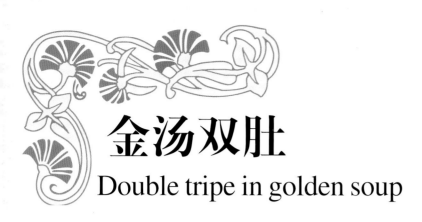

金汤双肚
Double tripe in golden soup

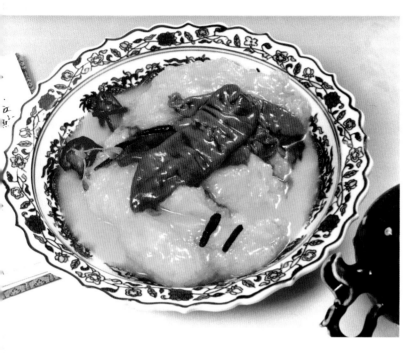

Main ingredient: 350g pan-fried Guang Du tripe, 150g soaked eel tripe.

Subsidiary ingredient: 5 piper longums, 0.2g red ginseng, 400g high-grade dense soup.

Flavouring: 6g zinc salt, 4g fresh sauce, 2g chicken oil, 100g fruit of Chinese wolfberry sauce.

Processing:

(1) Roast the Guang Du tripe and red ginseng together until they become dense, then put them in a plate.

(2) Braise the eel tripe, red ginseng and fruit of Chinese wolfberry together until they become soft, then pour them over Guang Du tripe.

Characteristic: The shape of Guang Du tripe is yellow with moisture. The eel tripe is red and bright. This dish is absolutely delicious.

主料：油发广肚350克，水发鳗鱼肚150克。

辅料：毕菝5根，红参0.2克，高级浓汤400克。

调料：锌盐6克，鲜味汁4克，鸡油2克，枸杞汁100克。

制作：

(1) 广肚与红参同烤至浓垫底。

(2) 鳗鱼肚与红参、枸杞汁等同烧至软糯扒在广肚上即可。

特点：广肚黄润，鳗肚红亮，香鲜软滑。

营养简析：

　　鱼肚与红参、毕菝一同烹制具有温补脾阳，散寒温胃的功效。其中，红参含有多种人参皂甙、糖类、氨基酸、维生素、微量元素等，有增强高级神经活动的兴奋与抑制过程，能提高脑力劳动的效率和应激能力；还可以促进蛋白质的合成。

鲜橘柴把肚

Fresh orange faggot tripe

主料：水发鱼肚40克。

辅料：仙人掌25克，金橘10克，枸杞子2克。

调料：锌盐3克，麻油2克，味精粉1克，芥末油2克。

制作：

（1）油发鱼肚挤净水分去腥，切丝用芥末、盐等调料拌匀捆成柴把。

（2）金橘对开，仙人掌切片入味拌制装盘即可。

特点：清爽利口，色泽艳丽。

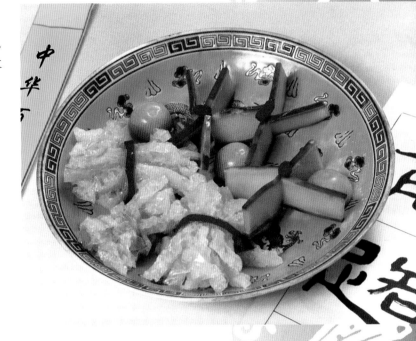

Main ingredient：40g soaked fish tripe.

Subsidiary ingredient：25g cacti, 10g orange, 2g fruit of Chinese wolfberry.

Flavouring：3g zinc salt, 2g seasame oil, 1g monosodium glutamate, 2g mustard oil.

Procesing：

（1）Eliminate the moisture of the deep—fried fish tripe and peculiar smell, cut it into shreds and bind it as faggot with mustard and salt.

（2）Cut the orange into the two pieces, cut the cacti into pieces and season them, then put them into a plate.

Characteristic：The taste is cleanlily and the color is flamboyant.

营养简析：

鱼肚与金橘一同烹制具有滋阴润肺，收敛阳气的功效。仙人掌与枸杞子中含有多量的黏性物质和多糖类物质，可起到保留人体内水分的作用。

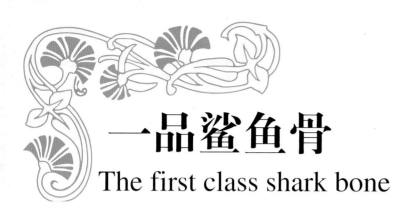

一品鲨鱼骨
The first class shark bone

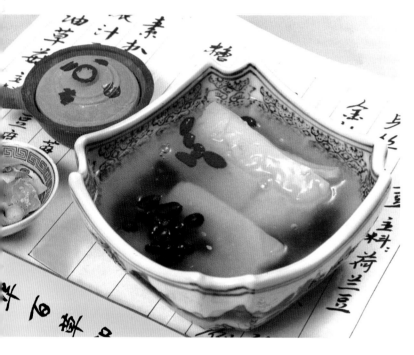

Main ingredient: 75g soaked shark bone.

Subsidiary ingredient: 15g black bean, 0.2g fruit of Chinese wolfberry, 200g high—grade clear soup.

Flavouring: 5g zinc salt, 4g fresh sauce.

Processing:

(1) After the bone is treated well, steam it with soup, black bean and fruit of Chinese wolfberry together for 40 minutes.

(2) Put the original sauce into the boiler and season it.

Characteristic: The sauce is clear and dense, the taste is salty and fresh. The original soup is seasoned with rich nutrition.

主料：水发鲨鱼骨75克。

辅料：黑豆15克，枸杞子0.2克，高级清汤200克。

调料：锌盐5克，鲜味汁4克。

制作：

(1) 鱼骨处理好后，入清汤加黑豆、枸杞子同蒸40分钟。

(2) 原汁入锅调好口味即可。

特点：汤汁清浓，口味咸鲜，原汤入味营养丰富。

营养简析：

鲨鱼骨中富含多量的软骨素，与含有多量多糖类物质的枸杞子及蛋白质含量丰富的黑豆一同烹制具有补肾利水、抗癌的功效。

茸菇鲨鱼骨

Pilose deer horn and mushroom cooked with shark bone

主料：鲨鱼骨50克。

辅料：鹿茸2片，草菇心50克，高级清汤250克。

调料：锌盐4克，火腿汁4克，瑶柱汁2克。

制作：

    (1) 鱼骨出水后加入清汤。

    (2) 鹿茸、草菇分别出水后，同鱼骨烧
          至汤汁浓稠，调味即可。

特点：味厚汁浓，醇鲜黏口。

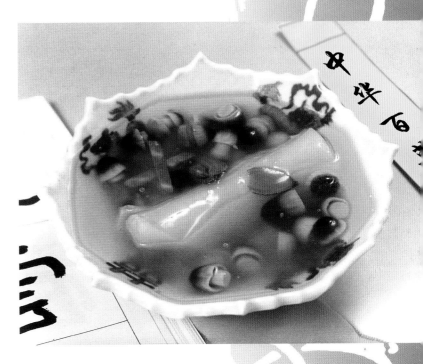

Main ingredient： 50g shark bone.

Subsidiary ingredient： 2 pieces of pilose deer horn, 50g mushroom, 250g high—grade clear soup.

Flavouring： 4g zinc salt, 4g ham sauce, 2g shellfish sauce.

Processing：

(1) After the fish bone is boiled lightly, put it into the soup.

(2) After the pilose deer horn and mushroom are boiled lightly in the water, braise them with fish bone together in soy sauce until the sauce becomes dense. Season it.

Characteristic： The taste is fragrant and the sauce is dense.

营养简析：

    鲨鱼骨与鹿茸一起烹制具有补脾肾，强筋健骨的功效。草菇中含有多种人体必需的氨基酸，对人体合成蛋白质有很大好处。

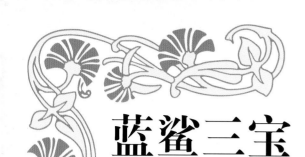

蓝鲨三宝

Three treasures of blue shark

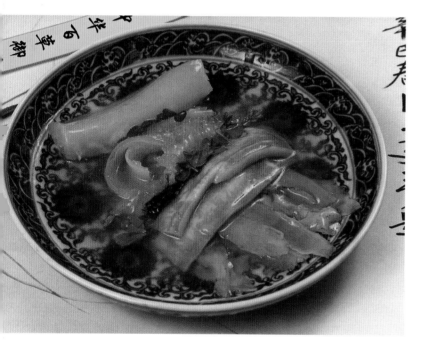

Main ingredient：25g shark bone, 25g shark skin, 25g shark lip.

Subsidiary ingredient：5g astraglus base, 10 granules of fruit of Chinese wolfberry, a little hair vegetable, 150g high—grade clear soup.

Flavouring：5g zinc salt, 3g monosodium glutamate, 1g pepper powder, 3g Shaoxing rice wine.

Processing：

(1) After the shark bone, shark skin and shark lip are soaked in the water, boil them lightly with Shao—xing rice wine to eliminate the peculiar smell.

(2) Hair vegetable, fruit of Chinese wolfberry and astraglus base are soaked separately.

(3) Put the main ingredients into the clear soup and steam them for about 40 minutes. Take out the original sauce and pour the starchy sauce over the dish.

Characteristic：It is fragrant with proper fire control and it is nourishing food.

主料：鲨鱼骨25克，鲨鱼皮25克，鲨鱼唇25克。

辅料：黄芪5克，枸杞子10粒，发菜少许，高级清汤150克。

调料：锌盐5克，味精3克，胡椒粉1克，绍酒3克。

制作：

(1) 鲨鱼骨、鲨鱼皮、鲨鱼唇分别水发后加绍酒出水，去腥异味。

(2) 发菜、枸杞子、黄芪分别水发。

(3) 经过处理后主辅料加入清汤中，上笼蒸40分钟左右，原汁倒出勾芡即可。

特点：鲜香浓郁，注重火候，滋补佳品。

营养简析：

鲨鱼骨、鲨鱼皮、鲨鱼唇中含有丰富的软骨素，及胶质蛋白及碘和多种矿物质。黄芪含有多糖、叶酸以及硒、锌、铜等微量元素，有保肝、利尿、抗衰老、降压和广泛抗菌以及调节血糖含量的作用。

荷花鱼骨
Lotus fish bone

主料：荷花雀13只。

辅料：鲨鱼骨100克，高级浓汤150克，杜仲 0.2克。

调料：锌盐8克，鲜味汁4克，鸡油2克，白 胡椒粒1克。

制作：

(1) 荷花雀腌入味后炸成金红色，出水 后与杜仲同蒸40分钟后装入盘中。

(2) 水发鲨鱼骨切成粒加胡椒粒与浓 汁烧制后扒在盘中即可。

特点：禽香四溢，色彩分明，口味咸香。

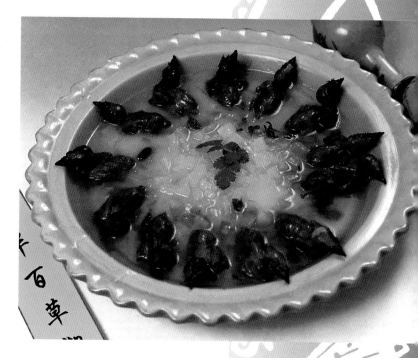

Main ingredient：13 lotus birds.

Subsidiary ingrdient：100g shark bone, 150g high-grade dense soup, 0.2g Eucommia ulmoides.

Flavouring：8g zinc salt, 4g fresh sauce, 2g chicken oil,1g white pepper.

Processing：

(1) After the lotus birds are pickled with flavouring, deep-fry them into golden and red color. Steam them with Eucommia ulmoides together for 40 minutes and put them into the plate.

(2) Cut the soaked shark bones into granules, put the pepper granules in, then braise it in soy sauce with dense sauce and pour it over the dish.

Characteristic：It is fragrant, the color is bright and the taste is salty fragrant.

营养简析：

鲨鱼骨与富含"硒"元素的禾花雀以及杜仲一起扒制，其中的软骨素与硒元素可起到强筋壮骨，清除体内衰老细胞的功效。其中，杜仲含有杜仲胶、杜仲甙、黄铜类以及鞣质等，有增强肾上腺皮质功能，增强机体免疫力功能和镇静、镇痛以及利尿的作用，还有较好的降压作用。

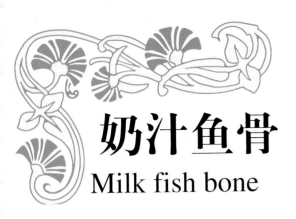

奶汁鱼骨
Milk fish bone

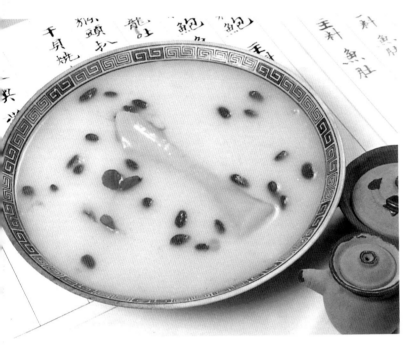

Main ingredient：65g soaked shark bone.
Subsidiary ingrdient：3g fruit of Chinese wolfberry, 150g high-grade milk soup. 2g bean seedling.
Flavouring：4g zince salt, 3g fresh sauce, 2g Shaoxing rice wine.
Processing：
(1) After the shark bone is boiled in water lightly, steam it in the soup.
(2) Season the milk soup and put the fruit of Chinese wolfberry in it and put the bones and seedling in to be boiled.
Characteristic：The soup is white and the bone is crystal and crisp.

主料：水发鲨鱼骨65克。
辅料：枸杞子3克，高级奶汤150克，豆苗2克。
调料：锌盐4克，鲜味汁3克，绍酒2克。
制作：
(1) 鱼骨出绍酒水后入毛汤蒸透。
(2) 奶汤调味加枸杞子等烧开下入鱼骨、撒豆苗即可。
特点：汤汁洁白，鱼骨透明爽脆。

营养简析：
　　鱼骨中含有鱼骨素等多种抗癌物质。奶汤中含有多种必需氨基酸，易于人体合成蛋白质。与枸杞子三者结合具有益寿助生的功效。

花果驼峰
Fig hump

主料：驼峰150克。

辅料：无花果10粒，枸杞子0.2克，浓汁100克，豆苗少许。

调料：碘盐6克，火腿汁5克。

制作：驼峰初步处理好后，入清汤与无花果、枸杞子同燉至软烂，入味勾汁撒豆苗即可。

特点：咸香回甜，软烂适口。

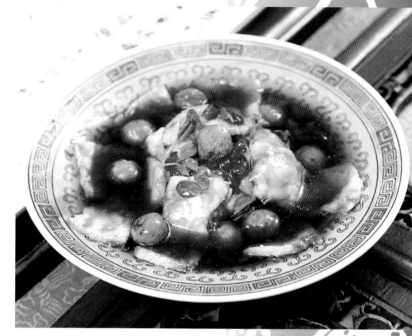

Main ingredient：150g hump.

Subsidiary ingredient：10 granules of fig, 0.2g fruit of Chinese wolfberry, 100g dense sauce, a little bean seedling.

Flavouring：6g iodin salt, 5g ham sauce.

Processing：After the hump is treated well, put it into the soup and braise it in soy sauce with fig and fruit of Chinese wolfberry together until it is soft. Season it and pour the starchy sauce over the dish and put the bean seedling on it.

Characteristic：The taste is salty fragrant and the meat is soft.

营养简析：

　　驼峰中含有丰富的胶质，脂肪，无花果中所含有的消化酶有利于胶质，脂肪的分解成氨基酸、脂肪酸，有利于人体的吸收。

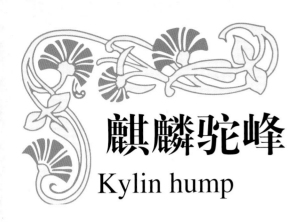

麒麟驼峰
Kylin hump

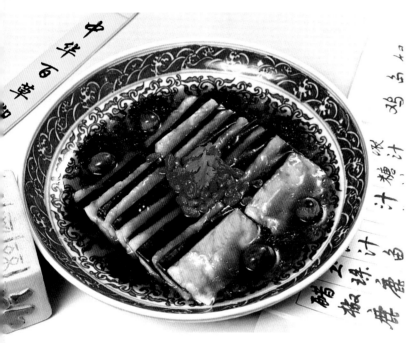

Main ingredient：250g hump.

Subsidiary ingredient：100g soaked kelp, 1g Amomum tsao-ko juice, 10g fruit of Chinese wolfberry, 100g high-grade soup.

Flavouring：10g iodin salt, 6g ham sauce, 2g pepper powder, 2g shallot oil.

Processing：

(1) Cut the soaked hump into pieces.

(2) Cut the kelp into pieces and make the kelp pieces and hump become kylin shape.

(3) Pour the soup and put a little Amomum tsao-ko into the soup and steam them with fruit of Chinese wolfberr together.

Characteristic：The shape is like kylin, the taste is fragrant and fresh with soft feel.

主料：驼峰250克。

辅料：水发海带100克，草果汁1克，枸杞子10克，上汤100克。

调料：碘盐10克，火腿汁6克，胡椒粉2克，葱油2克。

制作：

(1) 发好的驼峰切成排骨片。

(2) 海带去腥后切片与驼峰叠成麒麟状。

(3) 加上汤入草果汁少许，与枸杞同蒸即可。

特点：形似麒麟，味道香鲜，口感软烂。

营养简析：

驼峰与海带、枸杞子一同烹制具有补脾肾，消瘿瘤的功效。海带中含有丰富的碘对于单纯性甲状腺肿有很好的治疗作用。

香麻驼峰
Fragrant sesame hump

主料：驼峰 50 克。

辅料：芝麻仁 10 克，熟地黄 0.1 克。

调料：碘盐 4 克，胡椒粉 2 克，绍酒 2 克。

制作：

(1) 发好的驼峰切成片状，腌入味。

(2) 炒好的熟地黄磨成粉后沾在驼峰上，再沾蛋液及芝麻。

(3) 油 160 摄氏度左右下入，炸至外焦里嫩即可。

特点：麻香扑鼻，外焦里嫩。

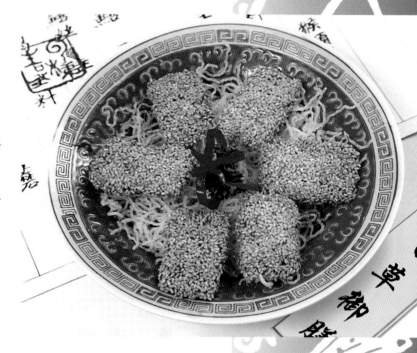

Main ingredient：50g hump.

Subsidiary ingredient：10g sesame, 0.1g prepared rehmannia root.

Flavouring：4g iodin salt, 2g pepper powder, 2g Shaoxing rice wine.

Processing：

(1) Cut the hump into pieces and pickle them with flavouring.

(2) Grind the cooked prepared rehmannia root and put it on the hump, the roll the hump in egg white and sesame.

(3) Deep-fry in 160℃ oil until it is burnt outside and tender inside.

Characteristic：The sesame is fragrant with burnt outside and tender inside.

营养简析：

　　驼峰与芝麻仁、熟地黄一同烹制具有补肾阳，润肠通便的功效。芝麻仁中含有多量的油脂（不饱和脂肪酸），有调节人体血脂代谢，润滑肠道的作用。

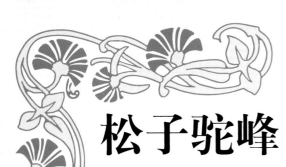

松子驼峰

Hump cooked with pine nut

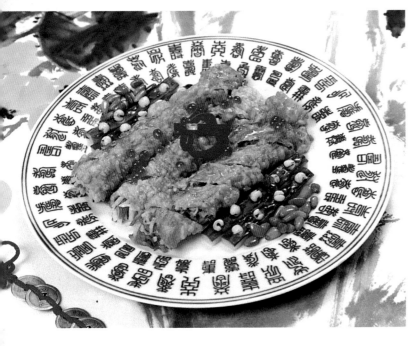

Main ingredient：50g hump.

Subsidiary ingredient：10g pine nuts, 5g red pepper shreds, 5g the seeds of Job's tears, 3g pieces of bean curd pieces, 2g roe.

Flavouring：6g iodin salt, 2g pepper powder, 2g Shaoxing rice wine.

Processing：

(1) Make the bean curd piece be soft in the water.

(2) Cut the soaked hump into shreds and season them.

(3) After seasoning the pine nuts, the seeds of Job's tears, roe and red pepper shreds, they are rolled with the hump into the bean curd piece and deep-fry the roll.

Characteristic：The bean curd piece is crisp, the hump is soft and the taste is fragrant.

主料：驼峰 50 克。

辅料：松子 10 克，红椒丝 5 克，薏米 5 克，腐皮 3 张，鱼籽 2 克。

调料：碘盐 6 克，胡椒粉 2 克，绍酒 2 克。

制作：

(1) 腐皮拍水使其回软。

(2) 发好的驼峰切成丝，拌入味。

(3) 松子、薏米、鱼籽、红椒丝等入味后与驼峰同卷入腐皮中炸制即可。

特点：腐衣酥脆，驼峰软烂，口味香浓。

营养简析：

驼峰与松子、鱼籽一同烹制具有温补脾肾，益肝血的功效。松子中含有多量的不饱和脂肪酸和维生素 A、维生素 D；鱼籽中含有丰富的蛋白质以及激素类物质，有抗衰老的作用。

合欢驼峰
Hump cooked with cortex albiziae

主料：驼峰 25 克。

辅料：芦荟 20 克，合欢皮 3 克，高级清汤 50
　　　克，枸杞子 0.2 克。

调料：碘盐 5 克，瑶柱汁 2 克，火腿汁 4 克，
　　　葱油 2 克。

制作：

（1）发制好的驼峰切片后与合欢皮、枸
　　　杞子同蒸 35 分钟。

（2）芦荟出水后与驼峰共同扒制即可。

特点：荤素搭配，脂多不腻。

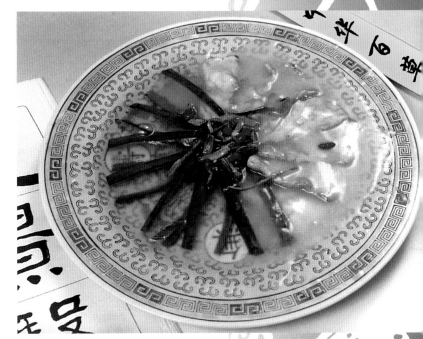

Main ingredient：25g hump.

Subsidiary ingredient：20g aloe, 3g cortex albiziae,
50g high—grade clear soup, 0.2g fruit of Chinese
wolfberry.

Flavouring：5g iodin salt, 2g shellfish sauce, 4g ham
sauce, 2g shallot oil.

Processing：

(1) Cut the soaked hump into pieces and steam
them with cortex albiziae and fruit of Chinese
wolfberry together for 35 minutes.

(2) After the cortex albiziae is boiled in water
lightly, cook it with the hump together.

Characteristic：More fat but it is not greasy with
meat and vegetable.

营养简析：

　　驼峰与合欢皮一同烹制
具有舒肝健脾、益肾阳的功
效。合欢皮还具有润肤美容，
保持青春的作用。

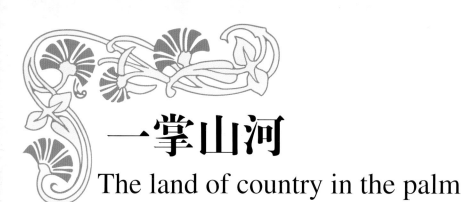

一掌山河

The land of country in the palm

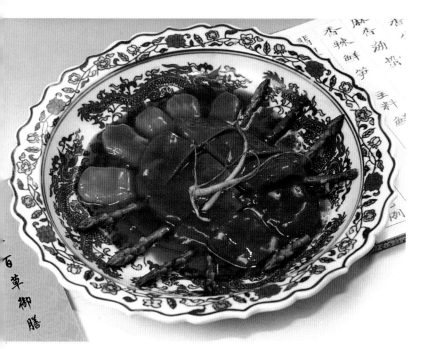

Main ingredient: 2 camel palms.

Subsidiary ingredient: 2g ginseng fiber and 30g fresh asparagus.

Flavouring: 4g Laochou flavouring, 6g Wanzi soy sauce, 4g sugar, 6g iodin salt, 6g Shaoxing rice wine.

Processing:

(1) After the camel palms are soaked well, season them and steam the ginseng fiber and the camel palms together for 40 minutes.

(2) After stir-frying the fresh asparagus, put it into a plate.

(3) Two camel palms are put together to shape them like bear palms.

(4) The original sauce is seasoned and pour it over the palms.

Characteristic: The shape is like bear palms, the color is red with moisture and taste is fragrant and soft.

主料：驼掌2只。

辅料：人参须2克、鲜芦笋30克。

调料：老抽4克，万字酱油6克，糖4克，碘盐6克，绍酒6克。

制作：

(1) 驼掌发好后，入味与参须同蒸40分钟。

(2) 鲜芦笋清炒后垫底。

(3) 两只驼掌对拼后码成熊掌状。

(4) 原汁调味扒在驼掌上即可。

特点：形似熊掌，色泽红润，香浓软烂，回味连绵。

营养简析：

驼掌与人参一同扒制具有补肾助阳的功效。鲜芦笋中含有丰富的膳食纤维以及维生素C和多糖类物质。

淮山扒驼掌

Huaishan yam cooked with camel palm

主料：驼掌 1 只。

辅料：鲜淮山 100 克，何首乌 0.1 克。

调料：老抽 3 克，料酒 6 克，万字酱油 3 克，
　　　白糖 2 克，干辣椒 2 克，香油 1 克，胡
　　　椒粉 2 克。

制作：

　　(1) 驼掌去骨入味与何首乌烧至软烂。

　　(2) 鲜淮山出水清炒垫入盘底。

　　(3) 驼掌原汁收浓即可。

特点：汁浓味重，咸鲜回辣，色泽红亮。

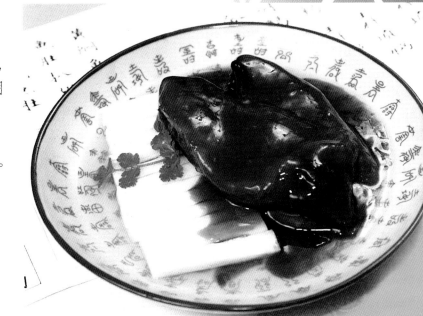

Main ingredient：1 camel palm.

Subsidiary ingredient：

Flavouring：3g Laochou flavouring, 6g flavouring wine,
3g Wanzi soy sauce, 2g sugar, 2g dry hot pepper, 1g
spiced oil, 2g pepper powder.

Processing：100g fresh Huaishan yam, 0.1g polygonum
multiflorum.

(1) The camel palm is boned and seasoned, then
braise it with polygonum multiflorum in soy
sauce until it becomes soft.

(2) Boil the fresh Huaishan yam lightly, then stir—fry
it and put it into a plate.

(3) The original sauce of the camel palm is boiled
until the sauce is reduced.

Characteristic：The sauce is dense, fresh and salty
with hot and red color.

营养简析：

　　驼掌与山药、何首乌一
同烹制具有补脾益精血的功
效。其中何首乌含有大黄
酚、大黄素、大黄酸等和羟
基蒽醌衍生物；并含卵磷
脂、鞣质，能促进红细胞生
成，增强免疫功能，降低血
糖；对心肌有兴奋作用，能
减慢心率，增加冠状动脉血
流；还可以降低胆固醇，减
轻动脉硬化。

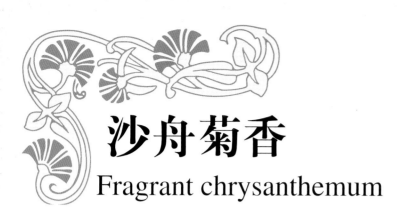

沙舟菊香
Fragrant chrysanthemum

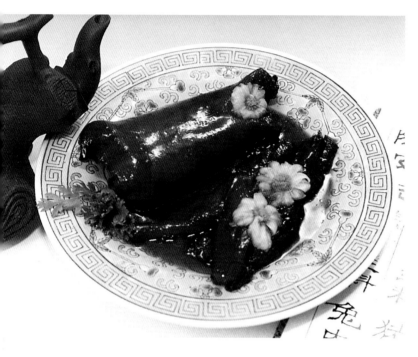

Main ingredient：300g camel palm, 150g camel tendons.

Subsidiary ingredient：2g dry chrysanthemum, 500g high—grade soup.

Flavouring：2g sugar color, 12g iodin salt, 4g granulated sugar.

Processing：

(1) After the camel palm and tendons are treated well, color them and deep—fry them.

(2) After coloring them, boil them until the sauce is reduced and put the chrysanthemum into the soup.

Characteristic：The color is red and bright, the taste is fragrant and the chrysanthemum smells good.

主料：驼掌300克，驼筋150克。

辅料：干菊花2克，上汤500克。

调料：糖色2克，碘盐12克，砂糖4克。

制作：

(1) 驼掌、驼筋经过初处理后上色过油。

(2) 上汤着色后入驼掌、驼筋等煲制，收汁前加入菊花即可。

特点：色泽红亮，口味香浓，菊香清远。

营养简析：

驼掌、驼筋与菊花一起煲制具有强筋壮骨，清肝明目的功效。其中菊花含有菊甙、黄铜类、维生素A样物质、维生素B_1，有镇静、解热作用，还有明显扩张冠状动脉的作用，菊甙有降压的作用。

玉翠驼掌
Jade camel palm

主料：驼掌1只。

辅料：西兰花25克，清汤50克，薏米5克，
黑豆2克。

调料：老抽3克，料酒6克，万字酱油6克，
白糖4克，碘盐6克，胡椒粉1.5克。

制作：

(1) 驼掌处理好后入味与黑豆、薏米
同烧至软烂。

(2) 西兰花清炒围在一侧。

(3) 驼掌拖出切成条，原汁调味扒在
其上即可。

特点：咸鲜回甜，原汁浓厚，软烂适口。

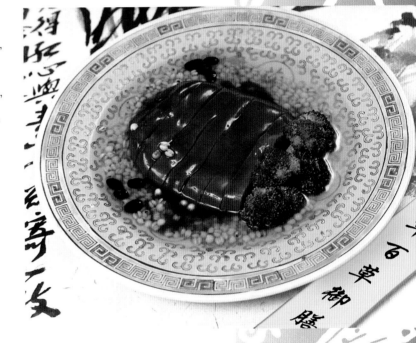

Main ingredient：1 camel palm.

Subsidiary ingredient：25g green cauliflower, 50g
clear soup, 5g the seeds of Job's tears, 2g black
beans.

Flavouring：3g Laochou flavouring, 6g flavouring wine,
6g Wanzhi soy sauce, 4g white sugar, 6g iodin salt,
1.5g pepper powder.

Processing：

(1) After the camel palm is treated well and seasoned,
braise it in soy sauce with black beans and the
seeds of Job's tears together until they are soft.

(2) Stir—fry the green cauliflower and put it aside.

(3) Take out the camel palm and cut it into loafs.
Pour the seasoned original sauce over the dish.

Characteristic：It is fragrant with salt, the original
sauce is dense and soft.

营养简析：

驼掌与薏米、黑豆一同
烹制具有健脾益肾，利水除
湿，强筋壮骨的功效。其中，
薏米、黑豆中含有赖氨酸、精
氨酸有助于人体合成蛋白
质，还有增强记忆力的作用。

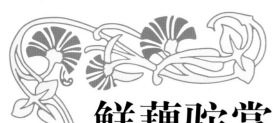

鲜藕驼掌

Fresh lotus root with camel palm

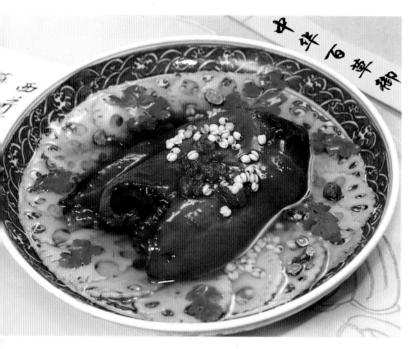

Main ingredient：1 camel palm.

Subsidiary：500g fresh lotus root, 3g Codonopsis pilosula, 3g the seeds of Job's tears, 2g fruit of Chinese wolfberry, 500g clear soup.

Flavouring：6g Laochou flavouring, 4g iodin salt, 6g Shengchou flavouring, proper quantity of the sugar, 25g Shaoxing rice wine.

Processing：

(1) After the camel palm is treated well, use boiled water to eliminate the peculiar smell.

(2) After rolling the camel palm in Laochou flavouring, deep—fry it in 180℃ oil to get color and put it into the soup and put Codonopsis pilosula, the seeds of Job's tears and fruit of Chinese wolfberry into the soup to be steamed together for 120 minutes. Then pour the starchy sauce over the dish.

(3) Peel the fresh lotus root and cut it into pieces and stir—fry them, then put them in the bottom of the plate.

Characteristic：The color is bright, the smell is fragrant and soft with sticky rice smell and rich nutrition.

主料：驼掌1只。

辅料：鲜藕500克，党参3克，薏米3克，枸杞子2克，清汤500克。

调料：老抽6克，碘盐4克，生抽6克，冰糖适量，绍酒25克。

制作：

(1) 驼掌经初步处理后，用开水去掉异味。

(2) 驼掌抹老抽后，油烧至180摄氏度左右下锅炸上色，入汤加入党参、薏米、枸杞子上笼蒸120分钟，后原汁入味扒制。

(3) 鲜藕去皮切片，清炒垫底即可。

特点：色泽明快，香浓糯软，营养丰富。

营养简析：

　　驼掌与鲜藕、党参、薏米、枸杞子一同烹制具有补益脾肾，利湿凉血的功效。驼掌中含有丰富的胶质蛋白；鲜藕中含有多量的黏蛋白。

龙马横空
Dragon and horse across the sky

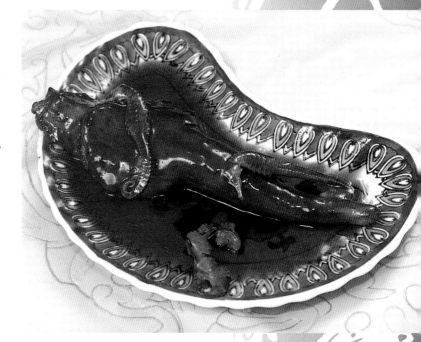

主料：鹿尾1只。

辅料：海马2只，高级清汤500克。

调料：生抽2克，糖色2克，美极鲜酱油6克，
冰糖5克，碘盐2克。

制作：

(1) 鹿尾去外皮烧毛后经出水等处理好。

(2) 海马用盐炒香。

(3) 鹿尾、海马同入清汤中蒸2小时
后，原汁入味调色烧至鹿尾软烂
即可。

特点：色泽红亮，软烂脱骨，胶质丰富。

Main ingredient: 1 tail of deer.

Subsidiary ingredient: 2 sea horses, 500g high—grade clear soup.

Flavouring: 2g Shengchou flavouring, 2g suger juice, 6g Meiji fresh soy, 5g rock sugar, 2g zinc salt.

Processing:

(1) After eliminating the skin of deer tail and fire the hair, use boiled water to treat it.

(2) Stir—fry the horse with salt.

(3) After steaming the deer tail and horses in the clear soup for 2 hours, braise the deer tail in soy sauce in the original sauce until it becomes soft with color.

Characteristic: The color is red and bright, the meant is boned and the colloid is rich.

营养简析：

鹿尾与海马一起蒸制具
有滋阴补肾的功效。海马含
有蛋白质、多种氨基酸以及
雄性激素样的物质可提高体
内的激素水平。

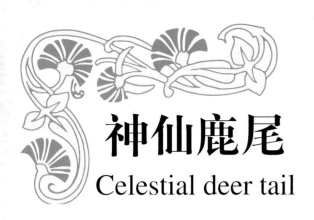

神仙鹿尾
Celestial deer tail

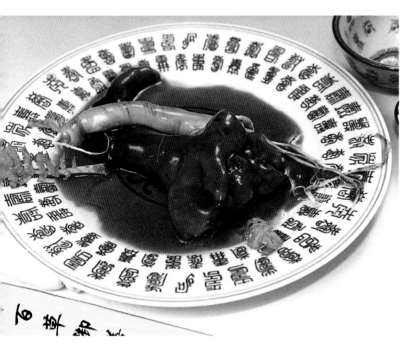

Main ingredient: 1 deer tail.

Subsidiary ingredient: 1 ginseng, 500g high-grade clear soup.

Flavouring: 3g Laochou flavouring, 3g granulated sugar, 8g salt, 2g pepper powder.

Processing: Eliminate the peculiar smell of the deer tail through boiling it lightly and deep-fry it to get color. Braise the ginseng in the soup for 3 hours to bone the deer tail.

Characteristic: The sauce is fragrant and the meat is soft. The color is golden and red and the taste is delicious.

主料: 鹿尾 1 只。

辅料: 人参 1 根，上汤 500 克。

调料: 老抽 3 克，砂糖 3 克，碘盐 8 克，胡椒粉 2 克。

制作: 将鹿尾初处理后出水去掉腥异味，过油上色。加上汤与人参燀3小时至鹿尾将脱骨即可。

特点: 汁香肉烂，色泽金红，口感丰富。

营养简析:

　　鹿尾与人参一同烹制具有补肾健脾，益智生津的功效。人参与鹿尾中所含的必需氨基酸的种类齐全，易于人体的吸收和利用。

益生双尾
Double tails for nourishing life

主料：马鹿尾2根。

辅料：口蘑6粒，素汤1000克。

调料：盐25克，老抽15克，鱼露18克，绍酒50克。

制作：

(1) 鲜鹿尾去毛，除异味。

(2) 入素汤、口蘑等同烧至将脱骨收汁勾芡即可。

特点：荤菜素汤，菇香清醇，肉香味浓。

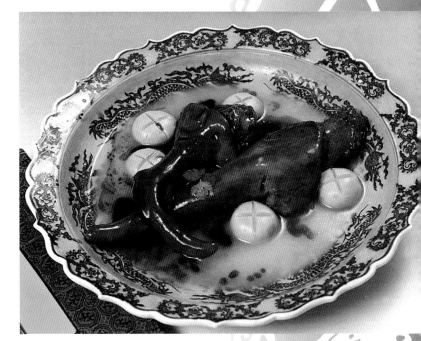

Main ingredient： 2 tails of red deer.

Subsidiary ingredient： 6 granules of mushroom，1 000g vegetable soup.

Flavouring： 25g salt，15g Laochou，18g fish sauce，50g Shaoxing rice wine.

Processing：

(1) Eliminate the hair of fresh deer tails, then eliminate peculiar smell.

(2) Put the vegetable soup and braise with mushroom together until they will be boned, pour starchy sauce over the dish.

Characteristic： It contains meat dishes and vegetable soup. The dish is fragrant mushroom with good wine. It is fragrant and savory.

营养简析：

　　马鹿尾与口蘑一同烹制具有补肾阳、益脾胃的功效。其中，马鹿尾中含有多量的蛋白质及胶质蛋白；口蘑中含有丰富的必需氨基酸，以及甘露醇和糖类物质。

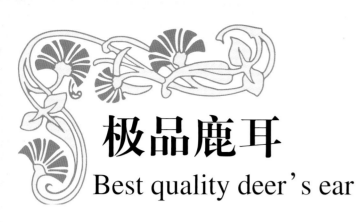

极品鹿耳
Best quality deer's ear

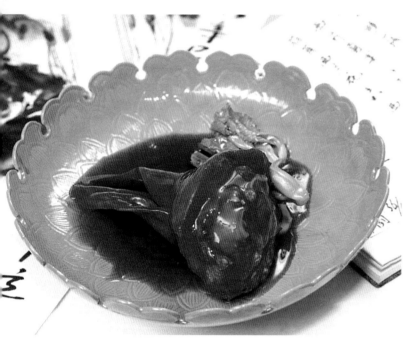

Main ingredient：One deer's ear.

Subsidiary ingredient：2g codonopsis pilosula, 500g old chicken, 500 pork sparerib, 10g Jinhua ham, 1 heart of leaf mustard.

Flavouring：6g Wanzi soy, 2g sugar juice, 6g iodate, 1 pepper, 3g granulated sugar, 1 000g Shaoxing rice wine.

Processing：

(1) Pickle the deer's ear for 4 hours after it is treated well.

(2) Braise the Codonopsis pilosula, old chicken, pork sparerib and ham in soy sauce together in Shaoxing rice wine for 3 hours until the original sauce becomes less, then put the dish in a plate.

(3) Stir—fry the leaf mustard.

Characteristic：The color is orange, the wine is fragrant, the bone is crisp and the meat is soft.

主料：鹿耳一只。

辅料：党参2克，老鸡500克，猪排500克，金华火腿10克，芥菜心1根。

调料：万字酱油6克，糖色2克，碘盐6克，辣椒1克，砂糖3克，绍酒1 000克。

制作：

(1) 鹿耳初处理后入味腌制4小时。

(2) 与党参、老鸡、猪排、火腿等同入绍酒中烧3小时后，原汁收浓入盘。

(3) 芥菜清炒即可。

特点：色泽橘红，酒香浓郁，骨酥肉烂。

营养简析：

鹿耳与党参一同烧制具有补肾聪耳，健脾益气的功效。其中党参含有皂甙、微量的生物碱、糖类、维生素B₁、维生素B₂，多种人体必需的氨基酸以及微量元素；能扩张周围血管而降低血压，又可抑制肾上腺素的升压作用；还可提高人体内的白细胞，增强抵抗力的作用。

杞米乌龙

Black dragon cooked with fruit of Chinese wolfberry and the seed of Job's tears

主料：乌参 1 只。

辅料：薏米25克，枸杞子10克，高级清汤50克。

调料：糖色3克，生抽4克，砂糖1克，麻油
1克。

制作：

(1) 乌参火发后，入汤与薏米、枸杞子
同蒸至软烂。

(2) 香葱起锅入乌参烧制。

(3) 薏米、杞子原汁调味浇在四周即可。

特点：色泽乌亮，口感软滑，口味咸香。

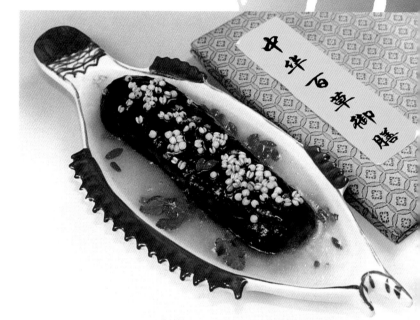

Main ingredient：1 black sea cucumber.

Subsidiary ingredient：25g the seeds of Job's tears,
10g fruit of Chinese wolfberry, 50g high—grade clear
soup.

Flavouring：3g sugar color, 4g Shengchou flavouring,
1g granulated sugar, 1g sesame oil.

Processing：

(1) After the black sea cucumber is quick—fried, put
it into the soup and steam it with the seeds of
job's tears and fruit of Chinese wolfberry until
it is soft.

(2) Put the shallot into the oil, then put the cucumber
into the boiler to be braised in soy sauce.

(3) The seeds of Job's tears and fruit of Chinese
wolfberry are seasoned with original sauce and
pour them around the cucumber.

Characteristic：The color is bright, the taste is soft
and fragrant with salt.

营养简析：

大乌参与薏米、枸杞子
一同烧制具有补肾益精，健
脾利湿的功效。乌参中含有
多量的烟酸（尼克酸），可起
到软化血管的作用。

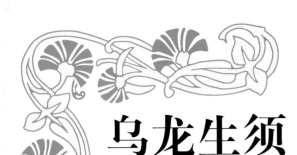

乌龙生须
The black dragon growing beard

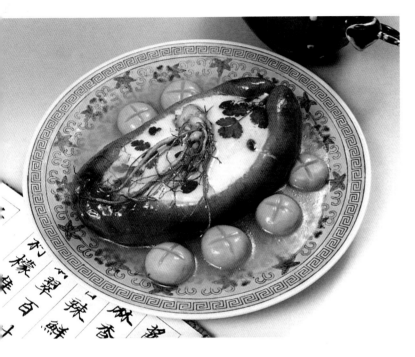

Main ingredient: 1 big sea cucumber.

Subsidiary ingredient: 1 ginseng beard, 50g chicken breast, 6 granules of mushroom, 50g high-grade soup.

Flavouring: 6g iodin salt, 8g fresh sauce, 6g chicken oil.

Processing:

(1) After the big sea cucumber is quick-fried, steam it with ginseng together.

(2) Make the chicken breast into fine and soft meat and it is pickled in soy sauce in the sea cucumber. Inlay the ginseng beard.

(3) Put the pickled sea cucumber into the soup and steam it with mushroom for 10 minutes, after that, pour the original sauce over it.

Characteristic: The color is bright, the taste is tender and salty fresh.

主料: 大乌参1只。

辅料: 人参须1根, 鸡胸肉50克, 口蘑6粒, 上汤 50克。

调料: 碘盐6克, 鲜味汁8克, 鸡油6克。

制作:

(1) 大乌参火发后与人参同蒸软。

(2) 鸡胸肉等制成茸酿入乌参中;镶入参须。

(3) 酿海参入汤与口蘑同蒸10分钟后, 原汁 浇上即可。

特点: 色泽明快, 口感软嫩, 口味咸鲜。

营养简析:

　　大乌参与人参一同蒸制具有补肾益精的功效。乌参与鸡胸肉、口蘑中必需氨基酸种类齐全, 易于人体的吸收。

乌龙吐珠

Black dragon spitting the pearl

主料：水发刺参 750 克。

辅料：鸽蛋 10 只，无花果 10 粒，上汤 50 克。

调料：糖色 4 克，生抽 3 克，砂糖 2 克，锌盐
 4 克，葱油 2 克。

制作：

（1）海参水发好后与无花果同用葱油烧。

（2）鸽蛋入浓汁烧后浇在四周即可。

特点：造型生动，黑白相衬，口味香浓。

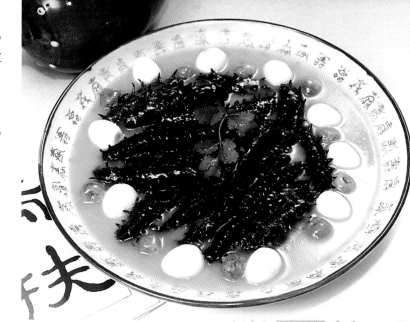

Main ingredient：750g soaked stichopus japonicus.

Subsidiary ingredient：10g pigeon eggs, 10 granules of fig, 50g high—grade soup.

Flavouring：4g sugar color, 3g Shengchou flavouring, 2g granulated sugar, 4g zinc salt, 2g shallot oil.

Processing：

（1）After the sea cucumber is soaked well, braise it in soy sauce and shallot with fig together.

（2）After the pigeon eggs are braised in the sauce, pour it around.

Characteristic：The shape is vivid with black and white colors and the taste is fragrant.

营养简析：

　　刺参、鸽蛋与无花果一同烹制，其中的蛋白质可被无花果中的消化酶分解为氨基酸，易于人体吸收。

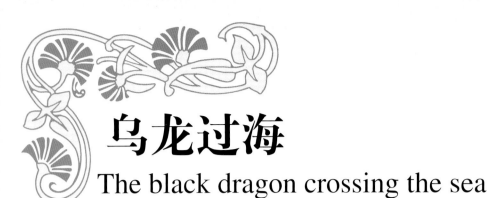

乌龙过海

The black dragon crossing the sea

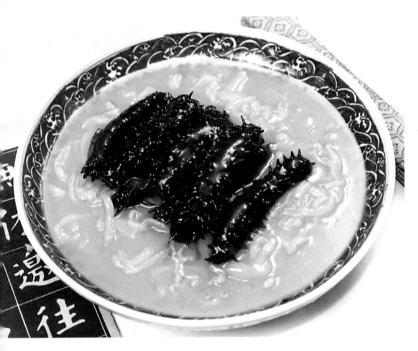

Main ingredient：250g soaked stichopus japonicus in water，250g jellyfish.

Subsidiary ingredient：3g Laochou flavouring，2g granulated sugar，5g Shengchou flavouring，1g mixed oil.

Processing：

(1) After the sea cucumber is treated well，braise it in soy sauce.

(2) Cut the jellyfish into shreds and boil them lightly. Put them into the seasoned dense sauce.

Characteristic：The shellyfish is crisp，the stichopus japonicus and the sauce is spiced.

主料：水发刺参250克，海蜇250克。

辅料：浓汤500克。

调料：老抽3克，砂糖2克，生抽5克，混合油1克。

制作：

　　(1) 海参初处理好后红烧。

　　(2) 海蜇洗净切丝出水，入调好的浓汁中即可。

特点：海蜇爽脆，刺参滑软，汁宽味足。

营养简析：

　　刺参与海蜇的蛋白质中的必需氨基酸种类齐全，还含有丰富的烟酸。二者一同烹制可起到补肾益精，降低胆固醇的功效。

益寿三宝
Three treasures of prolonging the longevity

主料：鹿鞭25克，鹿筋15克，鹿茸4片。

辅料：水发枸杞子0.1克，水发发菜0.1克，草菇心2粒，高级清汤100克。

调料：碘盐3克，鲜味汁4克，绍酒适量。

制作：

(1) 鹿鞭经处理去异味后剞刀出水使之成为鹿鞭花。

(2) 干鹿筋水发后使其吃足水分，回软。

(3) 鹿茸洗净。

(4) 将处理好的鹿鞭、鹿筋、鹿茸加枸杞子、发菜、草菇心入清汤调味同蒸40分钟即可。

特点：选料精细，原汁原味，清香可口。

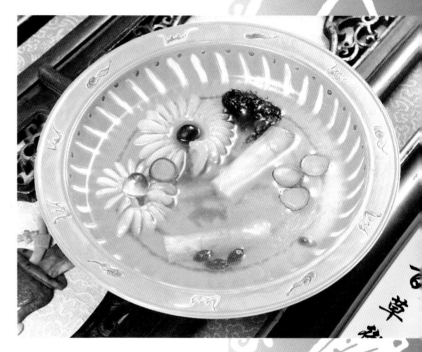

Main ingredient： 25g deer penis, 15g deer tendons, 4 pieces of pilose deer horn.

Subsidiary ingredient： 0.1g soaked fruit of Chinese wolfberry, 0.1g soaked hair vegetable, 2 granules of mushroom, 100g high—grade clear soup.

Flavouring： 3g iodin salt, 4g fresh sauce, proper quantity of Shaoxing rice wine.

Processing：

(1) After eliminating the peculiar smell of the deer penis, cut it and boil it lightly to make it become deer penis flower shape.

(2) After the dry deer tendon is soaked, make it absorb enough water to become soft.

(3) Clean the pilose deer horn.

(4) Put the deer penis, deer tendons, pilose deer horn, fruit of Chinese wolfberry, hair vegetable and mushroom into the clear soup to be seasoned and steamed for 40 minutes.

Characteristic： The ingredient is fine, the original sauce is fragrant and delicious.

营养简析：

鹿鞭、鹿筋与鹿茸枸杞子一同烹制具有补肾阳，强筋壮骨的功效，鹿茸中含有雄性激素、卵泡激素胶质、蛋白质、磷酸钙、碳酸钙等，有提高工作效率、减轻疲劳、改善睡眠和食欲、改善蛋白质和能量代谢的功效；以及增加红细胞、血色素、网织红细胞的作用；还能促进骨折的愈合。

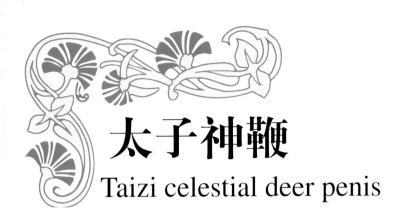

太子神鞭
Taizi celestial deer penis

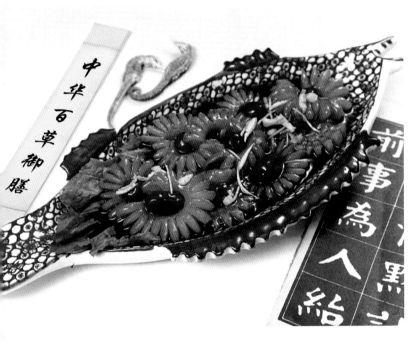

Main ingredient：750g fresh deer penis.

Subsidiary ingredient：0.3g Taizi ginseng, 5g Chinese dates.

Flavouring：4g Laochou flavouring, 3g iodin salt, 2g granulated sugar, 1g pepper powder, 4g Shaoxing rice wine.

Processing：

(1) Clean the fresh deer penis, boil it until the inner tube can be eliminated, then take it out.

(2) After eliminating the inner tube, continue to boil it until it becomes soft, then cut it into flower shape.

(3) Burn Chinese dates and eliminate the pits.

(4) Soak Taizi ginseng in water.

(5) Braise deer penis, Taizi ginseng, Chinese dates in soy sauce together until the deer penis becomes soft.

Characteristic：The color is red with moisture, the taste is soft with fragrant and sweet smell.

主料：鲜鹿鞭750克。

辅料：太子参0.3克，红枣5克。

调料：老抽4克，碘盐3克，砂糖2克，胡椒粉1克，绍酒4克。

制作：

(1) 鲜鹿鞭洗净，煮至可去内管，捞出。

(2) 去掉内管后，继续煮至软，后改刀成鞭花。

(3) 红枣烫过去核。

(4) 太子参用水发透。

(5) 鞭花、太子参、红枣入味同烧至鹿鞭软烂即可。

特点：色泽红润，口感软烂，口味咸香，回味微甜。

营养简析：

鲜鹿鞭与太子参、红枣一同烧制具有补肾益精、健脾补血的功效。太子参中含有果糖、皂武与富含蛋白质、糖类、有机酸、黏液质、维生素以及钙、磷、铁的红枣一同食用可起到保护肝脏、增加肌力、体力的作用。

天冬鹿脊髓

Deer marrow cooked with asparagus fern

主料：鹿脊髓250克。

辅料：天冬2克，黄精2克，高级清汤500克。

调料：碘盐4克，火腿汁3克，白胡椒粒1克，
    绍酒4克。

制作：

(1) 鲜骨髓，去水去异味杂物。

(2) 入清汤调味与天冬、黄精同蒸50
    分钟。

(3) 原汁入锅，调味收汁即可。

特点：口感松软，汁香味美，滋补佳品。

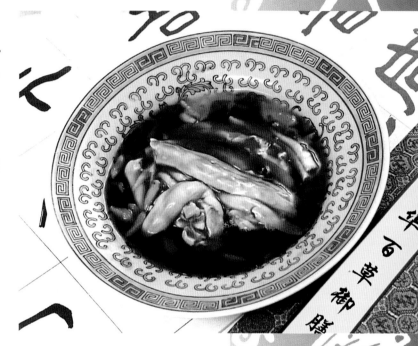

Main ingredient：250g deer marrow.

Subsidiary ingredient：2g asparagus fern, 2g seaswort,
500g high—grade clear soup.

Flavouring：4g iodin salt, 3g ham sauce, 1g white
pepper granules, 4g Shaoxing rice wine.

Processing：

(1) Eliminate the peculiar smell the water and impurity
    from the marrow.

(2) Put it into the clear soup and steam it with
    asparagus fern and sealwort together for 50
    minutes.

(3) Put the original sauce into the boiler, season it
    and reduce the sauce quantity by cooking.

Characteristic：It is soft and the sauce is delicious
and the dish is nourishing food.

营养简析：

　　鹿脊髓与天门冬、黄精
一同烹制具有补肾阴、益精
髓的功效。鹿脊髓中含有丰
富的卵磷脂，多食之对人体
的神经细胞可起到很好的补
养作用。

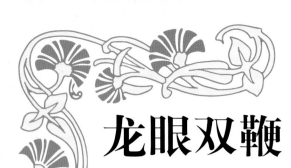

龙眼双鞭

Double deer penises cooked with longan

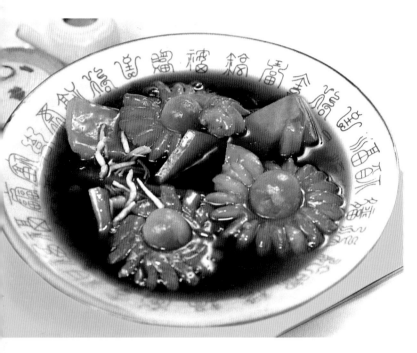

Main ingredient：50g deer penis, 50g qunbian.

Subsidiary ingredient：2g Taizi ginseng, 2g longan, 400g high—grade clear soup.

Flavouring：2g Laochou flavouring, 6g Meiji soy sauce, 3g iodin salt, 6g Shaoxing rice wine.

Processing：

(1) Boil the dry deer penis soaked to eliminate the peculiar smell, cut it in letter"one" word shape in China and boil it lightly to make it become chyssanthemum shape.

(2) Clean the soaked qunbian and put it into the clear soup with deer penis together, then put the Taizi ginseng in to be steamed together. After steaming, put the longan in it to season and color the dish.

Characteristic：The sauce is dense and spiced and the taste is like sticky rice smell.

主料：鹿鞭50克，裙边50克。

辅料：太子参2克，龙眼2克，高级清汤400克。

调料：老抽2克，美极酱油6克，碘盐3克，绍酒6克。

制作：

(1) 干鹿鞭水发后去异味，打成一字刀，出水，使其成为菊花状。

(2) 水发裙边处理干净，与鹿鞭同入清汤，加太子参蒸透后入桂圆调色调味即可。

特点：汤汁浓郁，口感软糯。

营养简析：

　　鹿鞭与裙边中含有丰富的动物胶，太子参中含有多糖、多种氨基酸和微量元素，能明显提高网状内皮系统的吞噬功能，提高免疫功能。龙眼中含有多种糖类如葡萄糖、蔗糖和维生素C、维生素B以及腺嘌呤、胆碱等成分。鹿鞭、裙边与太子参、龙眼一同烹制具有补肾滋阴，健脾益气，养心安神的功效。

红参鱼唇
Shark lip cooked with red ginseng

主料：鲨鱼唇 250 克。

辅料：红参 2 克，白芍 0.3 克，清汤 300 克。

调料：绍酒 10 克，锌盐 6 克，鲜味汁 4 克。

制作：

    (1) 鲨鱼唇水发后，入绍酒去水去异味。

    (2) 入清汤与红参同蒸 25 分钟。

    (3) 原汁调味即可。

特点：色泽洁白光亮，口感软烂，咸鲜适口。

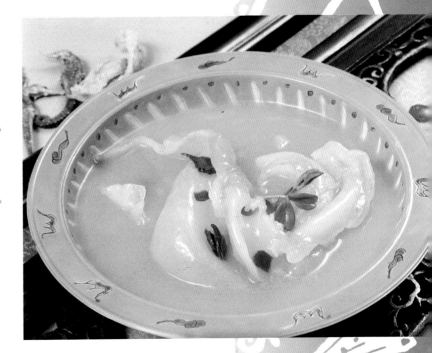

Main ingredient： 250g shark lip.

Subsidiary ingredient： 2g red ginseng, 0.3g root of herbaceous peony, 300g clear soup.

Flavouring： 10g Shaoxing rice wine, 6g zinc salt, 4g fresh sauce.

Processing：

(1) After the shark lip is soaked in water, put it into Shaoxing rice wine to eliminate the peculiar smell.

(2) Put it into the clear soup and steam it with red ginseng together for 25 minutes.

(3) Use original sauce to season.

Characteristic： The color is white and bright, the taste is soft and salty fresh.

营养简析：

    鲨鱼唇与红参、白芍一起烹制具有健脾舒肝的功效。白芍中含有芍药甙、鞣质树脂、牡丹酚可起到缓急止痛的作用。

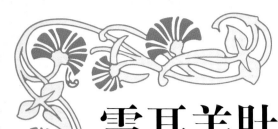

雪耳羊肚菌
Hickory chick cooked with tremella

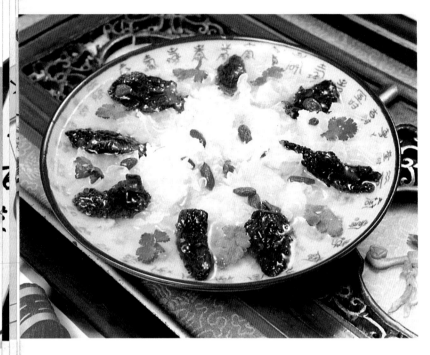

Main ingredient: 8 soaked hickory chicks.

Subsidiary ingredient: 20g soaked tremella, 1g fruit of Chinese wolfberry, 2g caraway, 250g high-grade clear soup.

Flavouring: 4g iodin salt, 10g fresh sauce.

Processing:

(1) Put the soaked hickory chicks into the soup and simmer them until they become soft.

(2) Put the tremella into the soup and steam it for 40 minutes.

(3) After the fruit of Chinese wolfberry is soaked in the water, the caraway is cleaned and put them on the dish.

Characteristic: The color is bright and clear and the taste is soft and sleek. It is good fungus food.

主料: 水发羊肚菌8个。

辅料: 水发雪耳20克, 枸杞子1克, 香菜2克, 高级清汤250克。

调料: 碘盐4克, 鲜味汁10克。

制作:

(1) 水发羊肚菌入汤煨至软烂。

(2) 雪耳入汤上笼蒸40分钟。

(3) 枸杞子水发香菜洗净, 消毒后点缀。

特点: 色彩分明, 口感软滑, 菌中佳品。

营养简析:

羊肚菌与银耳、枸杞子中含有丰富的多糖类物质, 具有很好的抗衰老功效。

红花双菌王
Saffron hickory chick king

主料：水发猴头菇 50 克，水发羊肚菌 6 只。

辅料：藏红花汁 10 克，胡萝卜 20 克，杞茸汁 5 克，高级清汤 100 克。

调料：碘盐 6 克，瑶柱汁 4 克。

制作：

(1) 羊肚菌发好后，入清汤蒸 40 分钟。

(2) 猴头菇浆好氽透，入清汤蒸 35 分钟。

(3) 胡萝卜切成十字架，出水。

(4) 高级清汤加入红花汁、杞茸汁调味后浇在菜品上即可。

特点：汤汁红润清澈，回味幽香。

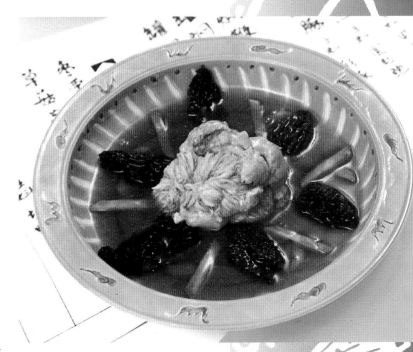

Main ingredient：50g soaked hericium erinaceus mushroom, 6 soaked hickory chicks.

Subsidiary ingredient：10g saffron sauce, 20g carrot, 5g fine and soft fruit of Chinese wolfberry sauce, 100g high-grade clear soup.

Flavouring：6g iodin salt, 4g shellfish sauce.

Processing：

(1) After the hickory chicks are soaked well, put them into the soup to be steamed for 40 minutes.

(2) After the mushroom is pickled and boiled, put it into the soup to be steamed for 35 minutes.

(3) Cut the carrot into Latin Cross shape and boil it lightly.

(4) Put the saffron sauce and fine and soft fruit of Chinese wolfberry seasoned into the soup and pour them over the dish.

Characteristic：The soup is red, clear and sleek with fragrant smell.

营养简析：

　　猴头菇与羊肚菌中的必需氨基酸的种类齐全，还含有丰富的多糖类物质，与活血祛瘀的藏红花一起烹制具有健脾舒肝，活血化瘀的功效。

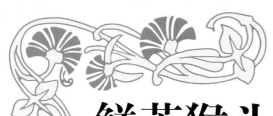

鲜芦猴头菇

Fresh aloe cooked with hericium erinaceus mushroom

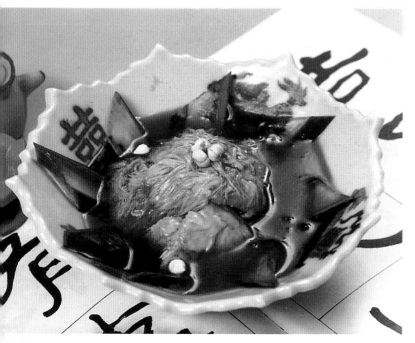

Main ingredient：2g dry hericium erinaceus mushroom．
Subsidiary ingredient：50g fresh aloe，2g the seeds of Job's tears，75g high—grade clear soup．
Flavouring：3g Laochou flavouring，4g iodin salt，3g fresh sauce．

Processing：

(1) After the dry hericium erinaceus mushroom is soaked，roll it in jam and boil it heavily．Put it into the soup to be steamed with the seeds of Job's tears until it becomes soft．

(2) Cut the fresh aloe into pieces，boil them lightly and stir—fry，then put the pieces around．

(3) Season and color the soup and pour it over the dish．

Characteristic：The color is red and sleek，the taste is salty and delicious with soft and sleek feel．

主料：干猴头菇2克。
辅料：鲜芦荟50克，薏米2克，高级清浓汤75克。
调料：老抽3克，碘盐4克，鲜味汁3克。
制作：

　　(1) 干猴头菇水发后，上浆余透，加汤上笼与薏米同蒸至透。

　　(2) 鲜芦荟切片出水清炒后码在四周。

　　(3) 高级清浓汤调色入味扒在其上即可。

特点：色泽红润，口味咸鲜，口感软滑。

营养简析：

　　猴头菇与鲜芦笋薏米一同扒制具有健脾利湿、抗肿瘤的功效。猴头菇、芦笋中含有丰富的多糖类物质，对癌细胞有很好的抑制作用。

双欢蛎皇
Double happy oysters

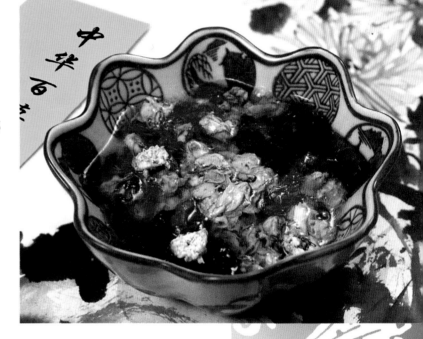

主料：鲜海蛎子 50 克。

辅料：藏红花 1 克，水发木耳 3 克，干菊花 0.5
　　　克，上汤 75 克。

调料：锌盐 4 克，胡椒粉 1 克。

制作：

　　(1) 鲜蛎皇原汤洗净。

　　(2) 红花、菊花入汤调味后下入蛎皇，
　　　　打沫即可。

特点：鲜味突出，菊香清心。

Main ingredient：50g fresh oysters.

Subsidiary ingredient：1g saffron, 3g soaked agaric,
0.5g dry chrysanthemum, 75g high-grade soup.

Flavouring：4g zinc salt, 1g pepper powder.

Processing：

(1) Clean the fresh oysters.

(2) After the saffron and chrysanthemum are put into
the soup and seasoned, put the oyster in it.

Characteristic：It is fresh and delicious with
chrysanthemum perfume.

营养简析：

　　蛎皇与藏红花、干菊
花、木耳一同烩制，具有清
肝明目，滋阴潜阳，通利肠
道的功效。蛎皇中含有丰富
的碘元素，对于单纯性甲状
腺肿有很好的预防作用。木
耳中含有多量的铁，多食之
会促进红细胞的生成。

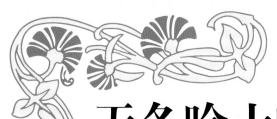

天冬哈士蟆

Fallopian tube of wood frog cooked with asparagus fern

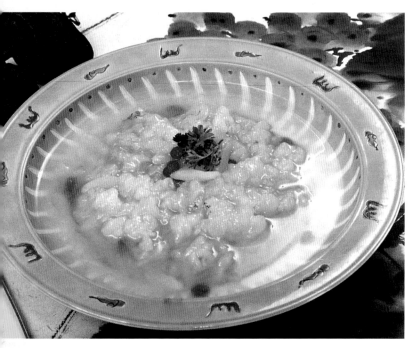

Main ingredient: 5g fallopian tube of wood frog.

Subsidiary ingredient: 1g asparagus fern, 1g fruit of Chinese wolfberry, 100g high—grade clear soup.

Flavouring: 6g zinc salt, 4g fresh sauce.

Processing:

(1) After the fallopian tube of wood frog is boiled, eliminate the peculiar smell and impurity.

(2) After the soup is seasoned, put fallopian tube of wood frog, asparagus fern and fruit of Chinese wolfberry into the soup to be steamed for 10 minutes.

Characteristic: The color is white like jade and the taste is delicious and soft.

主料：哈士蟆 5 克。

辅料：天冬 1 克，枸杞子 1 克，高级清汤 100 克。

调料：锌盐 6 克，鲜味汁 4 克。

制作：

(1) 哈士蟆水发后去杂质，除异味。

(2) 清汤调味后入哈士蟆、天冬、枸杞子上笼蒸 10 分钟即可。

特点：色泽如玉，鲜美滑软。

营养简析：

　　哈士蟆与天门冬、枸杞子一同烩制具有滋阴补肾的功效。对于潮热盗汗、骨蒸发热、阴虚火旺、虚火灼肺引起的咯血有很好的治疗作用。其中哈士蟆、枸杞子中含有多种激素类物质，以及丰富的多糖类物质，可以增强机体的免疫力。天门冬中含有黏液质、天门冬素具有抗炎、镇咳祛痰的作用。

雀鸟竹香
Birds stay with fragrant bamboo

主料: 鸽蛋 20 个。

辅料: 虾肉 75 克, 墨鱼肉 50 克, 鲜山药 100
克, 鲜竹叶 10 克, 清汤 250 克。

调料: 锌盐 6 克, 鲜味汁 6 克, 鸡油 2 克。

制作:

(1) 鲜山药切丝后炸成雀巢。

(2) 14 只鸽蛋过油, 烧制后入雀巢。

(3) 虾肉、墨鱼肉、鸽蛋制成 "小雀",
垫竹叶上笼蒸 6 分钟后扒汁即可。

特点: 造型活泼, 清鲜爽美。

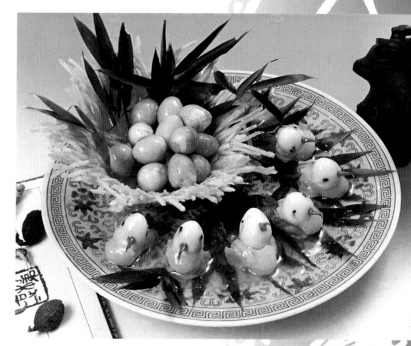

Main ingredient: 20 pigeon's eggs.

Subsidiary ingredient: 75g Shrimp, 50g cuttlefish,
100g fresh yam, 10g fresh bamboo leaves, 250g
clear soup.

Flavouring: 6g zinc salt, 6g fresh sauce, 2g chicken
oil.

Processing:

(1) After cutting the fresh yam into shreds, deep—
fried them to be the nest of the birds.

(2) Deep—fried 14 pigeon's eggs lightly, braise
them and put them in the nest of the birds.

(3) Make the young birds with shrimp, cuttlefish
and pigeon's eggs. Put the fresh bamboo leaves
on the bottom of the nest, then steam for six
minutes. Pour starchy sauce over the dish.

Characteristic: The sculpt is active. It is tasty and
refreshing.

营养简析:

鸽蛋与墨鱼、虾肉中的
氨基酸的种类齐全, 易于人
体合成蛋白质。与山药、竹
叶一同蒸制具有补肾健脾,
清心利尿之功效, 可以预防
消渴症。

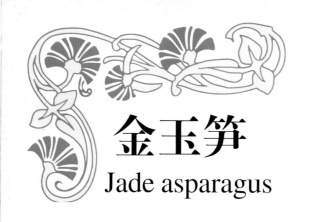

金玉笋
Jade asparagus

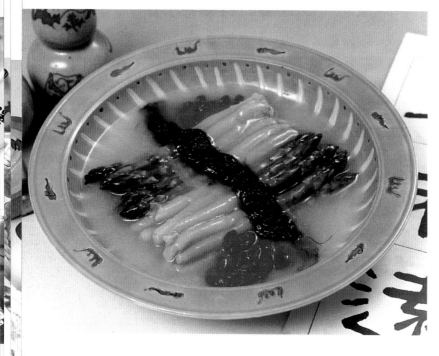

Main ingredient：100g fresh asparagus, 100g tin asparagus.

Subsidiary ingredient：3g hair vegetable, 4g fruit of Chinese wolfberry, 75g dense soup.

Flavouring：6g iodine salt, 4g shellfish sauce, 3g chick oil.

Processing：

(1) Fresh aloe and tin aloe are boiled separately.

(2) After the hair vegetable is soaked, eliminate the impurity and steam it in the soup with flavor.

(3) The fruit of Chinese wolfberry is soaked.

(4) Season the dense sauce and pour the starchy sauce over the dish with the chicken oil.

Characteristic：The color is bright, the sauce is fragrant and it smells spiced.

主料：鲜芦笋 100 克，罐装芦笋 100 克。

辅料：发菜 3 克，枸杞子 4 克，浓汤 75 克。

调料：碘盐 6 克，瑶柱汁 4 克，鸡油 3 克。

制作：

　　(1) 鲜芦笋、罐装芦笋分别出水。

　　(2) 发菜发透后去杂质，入汤蒸入味。

　　(3) 枸杞子水发。

　　(4) 浓汁入味勾芡，明鸡油，扒入即可。

特点：色泽明快，汤汁醇厚，口感丰富。

营养简析：

　　富含多糖的芦笋、枸杞子与矿物质含量丰富的发菜一起烩制具有健脾利湿、抗癌的功效。

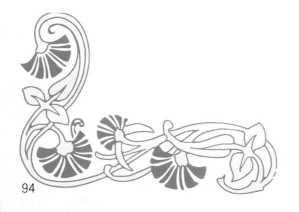

甘蓝鲜藕

Cabbage cooked with fresh lotus root

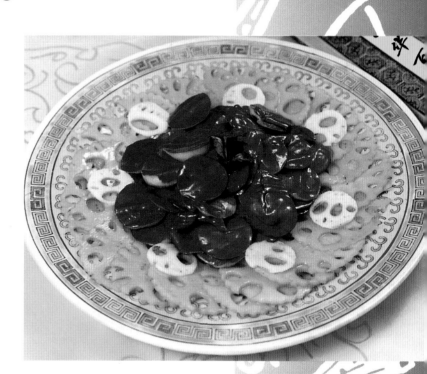

主料：紫甘蓝200克，鲜藕200克。

辅料：香菜少许。

调料：碘盐5克，柠檬汁25克。

制作：

  （1）甘蓝、藕分别切片。

  （2）藕用柠檬汁烧制，围在四周。

  （3）甘蓝清炒放在中间即可。

特点：色泽艳丽，清鲜爽口。

Main ingredient：200g purple cabbage, 200g fresh lotus roots.

Subsidiary ingredient：A little caraway.

Flavouring：5g iodin salt, 25g citric acid.

Processing：

(1) Cut the cabbage and lotus roots into pieces.

(2) Braise the lotus roots with citric acid and put them around a plate.

(3) Stir—fry the cabbage and put it in the middle of the plate.

Characteristic：The color is flamboyant and the taste is fresh and delicious.

营养简析：

  甘蓝与鲜藕中含有多量的维生素C、E以及丰富的黏蛋白，多食之可起到防治心血管疾病的作用。

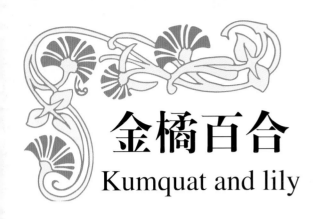

金橘百合
Kumquat and lily

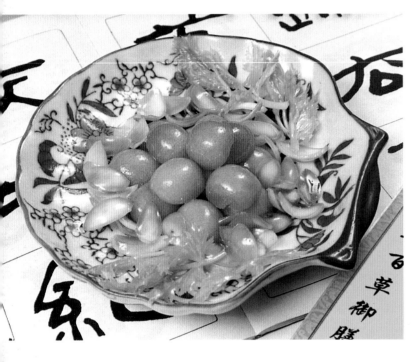

Main ingredient：250g kumquats.

Subsidiary ingredient：50g fresh lily, 25g celery.

Flavouring：6g iodine salt, 4g fragrant sauce.

Processing：

(1) Cut each kumquat into two halves, cut the lily into flower leaves and wash the heart of celery cleanly.

(2) When the temperature of the oil reaches about 150℃, oil the ingredients and stir-fry them.

Characteristic：The colour is terrific and the taste is delicious. To make sure the dish is done to a turn.

主料：金橘 250 克。

辅料：鲜百合 50 克，芹黄 25 克。

调料：碘盐 6 克，鲜味汁 4 克。

制作：

(1) 将金橘切成两半。百合切成瓣。芹黄心洗净。

(2) 油 150 摄氏度左右时，将原料过油后清炒即可。

特点：色鲜味纯，注重火候。

营养简析：

金橘与百合一同烹制具有滋阴生津的功效。其中金橘中含有多种有机酸，和橙皮甙有增强胃肠蠕动，排除胃肠积气的作用。百合中含有多种生物碱、淀粉等成分。

千层糕
Thousand layers cake

主料：玫瑰面粉300克。

辅料：咸鸭蛋黄2个，吉士粉3克，泡打粉1克，鲜酵母1克，黄油5克。

制作：面粉等和成发面团备用。把咸蛋黄蒸熟，搓碎加吉士粉拌匀。面团擀开，抹黄油、蛋黄一层一层做成千层糕。用牙签扎几下，醒发20分钟，蒸熟切件即可。

特点：口味甜香，口感软松。

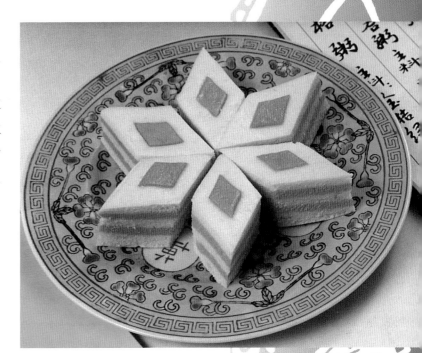

Main ingredient：300g rose flour.

Subsidiary ingredient：2 salty duck vitellines, 3g Jishi flour, 1g natron, 1g fresh yeast, 5g butter.

Processing：Put the flour and paste as standby. Steam the salty vitellines until they become ripe. Grind them and put Jishi flour in to be mixed together. Roll the paste in butter and vitellines on each layer to make thousand layers cake. Use the toothpick to prick it. Wait for 20 minutes, steam it and cut the ripe cake into pieces.

Characteristic：The taste is sweet, fragrant, soft and crisp.

营养简析：
　　玫瑰面中含有蛋白质、消化酶、脂肪酶、麦芽糖酶等多种消化酶，具有健脾消食的作用。咸蛋黄中含有多量的胆碱，对脑细胞有很好的补养作用。

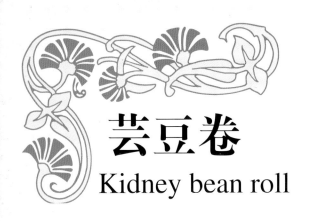

芸豆卷
Kidney bean roll

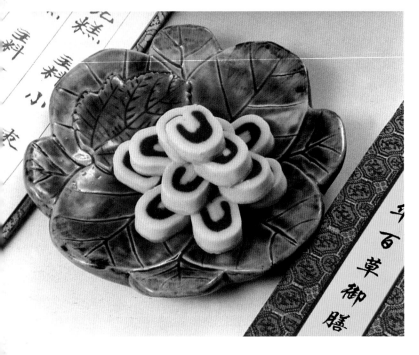

Main ingredient: 200g white kidney bean.

Subsidiary ingredient: 50g sweetened bean paste, 1g alkali flour.

Processing: Peel the kidney bean by soaking it with water and boil it. Put alkali flour in it for 20 minutes. After that, take it out and put it into the refrigerator after screenings. Stir the bean paste and take out the kidney bean flour and roll in the bean paste to be rolled. Cut it.

Characteristic: The shape is like Ruyi and the taste is cool and delicious.

主料：白芸豆200克。

辅料：豆沙50克，碱面1克。

制作：把芸豆用水泡软去皮，煮透。出锅出水过箩入冰箱备用。把豆沙调匀，取出芸豆面抹上豆沙卷起捏顺，切件即可。

特点：形似如意，口味清凉口感爽滑。

营养简析：

芸豆中含有丰富的蛋白质，其蛋白质分解后可产生多量的必需氨基酸。具有健脾利湿，益血补虚的功效。

御贡佛手
Imperial Buddha hand

主料：玫瑰面粉100克。

辅料：黄油40克，糖20克，豆沙30克，鸡蛋1个。

制作：

(1) 一半玫瑰面加水制成水油皮。

(2) 另一半加黄油制成油心。

(3) 水皮包油心制成酥皮，下剂包豆沙，制成佛手，刷蛋液烤制即可。

特点：形似佛手，皮脆陷软，口味甜香。

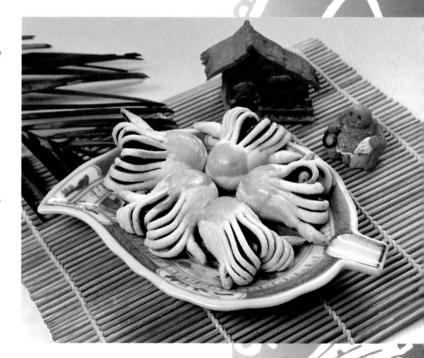

Main ingredient: 100g rose flour.

Subsidiary ingredient: 40g butter, 20g sugar, 30g bean paste, 1 egg.

Processing:

(1) Put the water into one half of the rose flour to make it into water oil peel.

(2) Put the butter into the another half to make it into oil center.

(3) Use the water oil peel to wrap the oil center to make crisp peel and put the bean paste in it to make Buddha hand. Put the egg liquid on it and roast it.

Characteristic: The shape looks like a Buddha hand, the peel is crisp and the stuffing is soft. The taste is sweet and fragrant.

营养简析：

　　玫瑰面中含有蛋白质消化酶、麦芽糖酶、脂肪酶等多种消化酶，有利于富含蛋白质、脂肪和糖类食物的消化。具有健脾消食的功效。

入膳药材的相关知识
The Relevant Knowledge of Herb-medicine Imperial Cuisine

党 参
Codonopsis pilosula

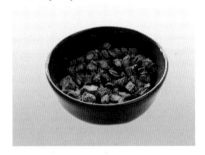

种属： 桔梗科党参。多年生草本，有白色乳汁。
产地： 主产于山西、陕西、甘肃、四川等地。
性味： 味甘，性平。
归经： 脾、肺。
功效： 补中益气，生津养血。
用途： 用于中气不足所致的食少便溏，四肢倦怠；还可用于肺气亏虚引起的气短咳喘，言语无力，声音低弱等症。热病伤津，气短口渴。以及血虚心失所养所致的面色萎黄，头晕心悸。
文献
摘录：《本草从新》："主补中气，和脾胃，除烦渴，中气微弱，用以调补，甚为平妥。"《本草纲目拾遗》："治肺虚，能益肺气。"

太子参
Taizi ginseng

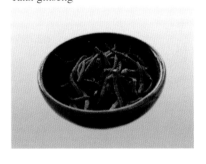

种属： 石竹科异叶假繁缕。多年生草本，高7～20厘米。块根纺锤形。
产地： 主产于中国江苏、山东、安徽等地。
性味： 味甘，微苦，性平。
归经： 脾、肺。
功效： 补气生津。
用途： 用于脾虚食少，倦怠乏力，心悸自汗，肺气虚所致的咳嗽，津亏口渴。
文献
摘录：《本草再新》中说："治气虚肺燥，补脾土，消水肿，化痰止咳。"

西洋参
American ginseng

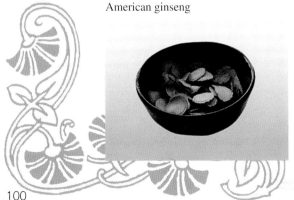

种属： 五加科西洋参。多年生草本。
产地： 原产于北美洲，中国东北、华北等地多有引进。
性味： 味苦，性微寒。
归经： 心、肺、肾。
功效： 补气养阴，清火生津。
用途： 用于阴虚火旺，虚火灼肺所致的喘咳咯血；热病及中暑气阴两伤，烦倦口渴；还可用于津液不足引起的口干舌燥等症。
文献
摘录：《本草从新》中说："补肺气降火，生津液，除烦倦。虚而有火者相宜。"《本草再新》中也有这样的记载："治肺火旺，咳嗽痰多，气虚咳喘，失血劳伤，固精安神。"

种属：豆科膜荚黄芪。多年生本草。

产地：主产于中国山西、黑龙江、内蒙古等地。

性味：味甘，性微温。

归经：脾、肺。

功效：补气升阳，益卫固表，托毒生肌，利水退肿。

用途：用于脾肺气虚或中气下陷所致的食少便溏，气短乏力，内脏脱垂（胃下垂、子宫脱垂）；气虚不能摄血所引起的崩漏、便血；还可用于卫气虚所致的表虚自汗；也可用于阴虚引起的盗汗；气血不足所致的疮疡久溃不敛；以及气虚失运，水湿停聚引起的肢体面目浮肿，小便不利，和气虚血滞导致的肢体麻木、关节疼痛或半身不遂等症。

文献
摘录：《本经》："主痈疽久败创，排脓止痛，大风痫疾，五痔鼠瘘，补虚，小儿百病。"

黄 芪
Astraglus base

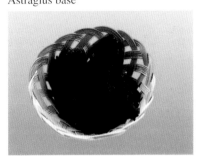

种属：薯蓣科薯蓣。多年生缠绕性本草。

产地：中国河南等省。

性味：味甘，性平。

归经：脾、肺、肾。

功效：益气养阴，补肺脾肾。

用途：用于脾虚气弱所致的食少便溏或泄泻；还可用于肺虚之喘咳；也可用于肾阳虚导致的遗精、尿频、妇女白带过多。此外还可用于消渴症，可补气养阴而止渴。

文献
摘录：《本草纲目》："益肾气，健脾胃，止泻痢，化痰涎，润皮毛。"《日华子本草》："主泄精，健忘。"

山 药
Yam

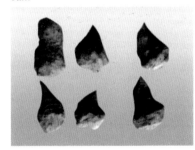

种属：百合科黄精。多年生草本。

产地：主产于河北、内蒙古、陕西等地。

性味：味甘，性平。

归经：脾、肺、肾。

功效：滋阴润肺，补脾益气。

用途：用于肺虚燥咳；肾虚精亏导致的腰酸、头晕、足软；以及脾胃阴虚所致的口干食少、饮食无味、大便干燥、似饥而不欲食。

文献
摘录：《别录》："补中益气安五脏。"《本草纲目》："补诸虚，填精髓。"

黄 精
Sealwort

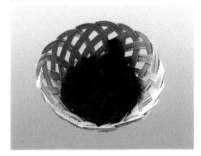

种属：麦角菌科冬虫夏草菌。

产地：主产于四川、西藏、青海等地。

性味：味甘，性温。

归经：肾、肺。

功效：益肾补肺，止血化痰。

用途：用于肾阳不足导致的阳痿遗精、腰膝酸痛；以及久咳虚喘，痨嗽咯血；还可用于病后体虚不复或自汗畏寒等症。

文献
摘录：《本草从新》："保肺益肾，止血化痰，已痨嗽。"《药性考》："秘精益气，专补命门。"

冬虫夏草
Cordyceps sinensis

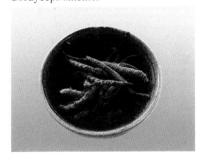

厘米，二年生的4～5厘米，10厘米以上的个头，大约要生长5～6年。鲍鱼在岩石上的附着力很强，它能忍受大浪的冲击，一个15厘米的鲍鱼，就有二百公斤的附着力，捕捉时最好不要惊动它，否则不易捕捉。

鲍鱼的种类很多，分布也很广，几乎全世界几大洋都有出产。日本、美国、墨西哥等国出产的鲍鱼都很好，特别是墨西哥的鲜鲍鱼，个大质嫩，被誉为"墨鲍"。干鲍鱼一般以日本产的为好。我国广东、山东、辽宁、台湾等地也有出产。

鲍鱼中的营养物质主要含有：蛋白质40%、脂肪0.9%、无机盐7.9%、糖33.7%，还较多的钙、铁、碘和维生素A、B、C等。

鲍鱼可以红烧、煲制、白扒、汆汤等，鲜鲍可油炸或拌食等。

鲍鱼贝壳可入药，名为"石决明"，有明目祛障的功效。还能清热、平肝、息风。

传统鲍鱼涨发方法：

多用水发，方法是：鲍鱼先用温水浸泡洗净，而后用热水浸泡12～15小时左右（水温保持在80～90度）捞出，入开水锅中文火煮2～4小时后，加入硼砂（一斤干鲍鱼加硼砂50克），焖泡10小时左右（水温仍保持在80～90度），而后用手捏鲍鱼，见已发透硬心，而且有弹力，捞出洗净，再用开水反复焯后（吐硼砂）即可蒸制使用。

鲍鱼涨发另一方法：

将鲍鱼洗净，入70～80度的热水中浸泡4小时，而后换清水加热（一斤干鲍鱼加硼砂20克），用文火煨煮2～4小时，离火后，继续在热水内浸泡（最好保持恒温70～80度），第二天换清水仍以文火煮两小时，至鱼体无硬心，有弹力，表里弹性程度一样即成。而后用开水反复焯后，即可烹制。

出成率：一斤干鲍鱼水发后一般出2斤半至3斤不等。

现在干鲍鱼或鲜鲍鱼的涨发一般采取煲制。十分讲究方法。原汁原味，一气呵成。

鱼 翅

鱼翅是鲨鱼的鳍干制成的。鲨鱼个体较大，捕捞较难。但是，捕捞史却相当古老。广东潮安的贝丘遗址发现为数极多的鱼骨，有些鱼的脊骨相当大，估计属于鲨鱼类。以此计算鲨鱼捕捞史已有四千年以上了。

一般餐饮业使用的鱼翅，是鲨鱼的鳍经过干制

而成的，鳍按其生长的部位，可分为背鳍、胸鳍、臀鳍、尾鳍。以背鳍制成的叫脊翅、背翅或劈刀翅、披刀翅、刀皮翅，呈三角形，翅多肉少，质量最好。以胸鳍制成的叫翼翅或上青翅、大青翅，呈三角形，一面凹，翅少肉多，质量较次。以尾鳍制成的叫尾翅，勾尖或发电勾。以臀鳍制成的称为荷包翅，翅根。尾翅和臀翅肉最多，翅最少，所以后两种翅的质量最差。

鱼翅按颜色分：有黄、白、灰、青、黑、混合等六种，其中以黄、白、灰色的质量较优。

由于产地和焙制方法不一，又有淡水干制法和咸水干制法之分，淡水干制的鱼翅用日光晒或用石灰水浸泡晒凉而成的，质量较好。咸水翅用盐水浸泡晒凉而成，质量次于淡水翅。

鱼翅还可按形状是否完整分类，涨发后成为整只翅的称为排翅，为上品。涨发后散开成一条一条的叫散翅、翅针。

一般来看鱼翅的种类有：

1. 肉翅（黄肉翅）

这种鱼翅中有一层像猪肥膘一样的肉，翅筋层层排在肉内，所以称为肉翅，这种鱼翅胶质丰富，质量较好。

2. 明翅，又名金花翅

明翅发透后成为一条一条散开的明翅，其质量仅次于肉翅。

3. 荷包翅

荷包翅是以小鲨鱼的鳍或其他鲨鱼臀鳍制成的。国家传统称为三连小鲨翅，皮落，翅筋细短，质地鲜嫩，次于金花翅。

4. 皮针翅

皮针翅是以划水鳍或尾鳍的外围生长的针形的鳍制做而成的。

鱼翅的产地：

我国鱼翅的产地主要在广东、福建、浙江、山东、海南、台湾等省。日本、美国、印度尼西亚、越南、菲律宾、泰国等国家均产，一般来说，进口鱼翅以菲律宾的吕宋黄即黄肉翅为佳品。国产的以台湾的大鲑口翅为最好（台湾海峡有鲨场）。

鱼翅以热带产的最好，温带产的鱼翅与热带相似。其中灰色质量较差。寒带的鱼翅，大都为青色，质量最差。

鱼翅的品质在外表上观察，疵点少的较好，但内部的质量却有出入，在检查鱼翅质量时必须注意以下五个方面：

1. 弓线色：鱼翅的形状很大，青黑色，淡性，翅筋细软而糯可能是中间有细长芒骨，不能食用。但可

将芒骨除去做散翅，仍为上品翅。

2．石灰筋：鱼翅的形状很大，青黑色，淡性，翅筋较粗，中间段发白，食之坚如灰石，不能下咽，因此，这种鱼翅饮食业不能使用。

3．熏板：它是冬季产的鱼翅，因无法用日光晒干，所以用碳火焙干，这种鱼翅在泡发时，外面的沙粒很难清除。必须细心去掉沙粒，由于质地坚硬，色泽不鲜艳，故称熏板。

4．油板：翅形大小都有，因为是成体，在阴雨季节，气候潮湿，由于产地未及时注意保管，刀割处的肉发生腐烂，影响到翅根部，呈紫红色，这一段地方腥臭异常，必须切除才能使用，在鉴别时，见到鱼翅根部似干非干，有油浸的现象，这就是油根的毛病，出现这种情况较少，但也应注意。

5．夹沙：是肉夹筋的白色鱼翅，在捕获时不慎压迫外皮，使沙粒陷入鱼翅的内部，晒干后即有深形皱纹。在泡发时用做排翅，沙粒很难取出，只有不惜耗损，拆开鱼翅，洗净沙粒，然后整成排翅。

涨发鱼翅时应先将鱼翅大小老嫩分开发制，以防发制时出现透烂不一致的现象。发好的鱼翅忌用铜、铁器盛装，以防变色。

涨发鱼翅时先用剪刀剪去鱼翅周围的毛边及脏物，而后用净水洗去尘土，放入盆内加温水浸泡10小时左右，再入锅用文火煨煮3～5小时左右，端离火口盖严闷泡5～6小时（水温保持在80度左右为好），见沙粒漂起，用手搓，小刀刮，去净表面沙粒，剪去鱼翅肉质腐烂的部位，剔净翅骨，用净水反复漂洗干净，而后码入碗内，加入好汤、葱、姜、大料，上屉蒸制翅筋软烂后取出，便可烹制。

出成率：上等鱼翅一斤出一斤或一斤二两左右。次等鱼翅一斤出六两至八两不等。

涨发鱼翅的注意事项：

1．涨发时忌用铜、铁容器，如用铜铁容器，鱼翅本身会起化学变化，出现黄色斑点，影响质量。最好用陶瓷器皿。

2．将鱼翅大小老嫩分开涨发，以免在涨发时，老的发不透，嫩的已发老。

3．容器不能沾有矾、碱、盐、油四种物质，否则会影响质量。

4．操作要细心，不要把鱼翅弄碎、弄断，影响出品质量。

5．去沙一定要干净彻底。

海 参

海参——海中人参，又名海鼠。它是一种棘皮动物，体呈圆柱形，前端有口极，口周围有触手，后有反口极（肛门），有感觉功能。海参的繁殖又称为"放浆"，是从背部放射出一股白色雾状物质，即精子或卵子，受精后产生耳状幼体，而后变态发育成幼参，它由浮游变成底栖，开始附在水底生活。披着褐黑色或苍绿色的外衣，身长着许多突出的肉刺，这就是海参。

海参的营养丰富，据《本草纲目》记载：海参有补肾、补血和治疗溃疡等疾病的效用。每百克海参含蛋白质61.6克，脂肪0.9克，碳水化合物10.7克，矿物质19.4克，含碘3000微克。所以它是一种优良的滋补品。

海参分有刺和无刺两大类：

有刺参包括：刺参、梅花参、黄玉参、辽参、广参、瓜皮参、大乌参、方刺参、十番参、九番参。

光参类：茄参、乌虫参（香参）、白石参、白瓜参（地瓜参）、克参（乌狗参）、乌乳参。

我国沿海海洋的食用海参有几十种，下面就简单介绍几种：

刺参（灰参）：

刺参个头不大，但体壁肥厚，肉质细糯，皮薄，它产于山东沿海和辽东半岛沿海，生活在海流较稳定的海湾内，喜栖于3～15米的岩礁或细泥沙的海底。它的身体背部布满大小不等的圆锥状肉刺，故名刺参。

海参既没有快速游泳的本领，又无强而有力的武器，惟一的法宝是"分身术"。当它受到刺激时，能将一部分内脏从肛门排出来。这是一种黏稠状的物质，用以迷惑敌人，而真身借机避开敌害。海参失去这部分内脏还可以重新长出来。海参不但能重新长出失去的内脏，而且还能长出身体的其他部分。若把海参切成两半放回海里，经过三四个月，分开的头尾又能重新长成新海参，再生能力较强。海参生长适宜的水温为3～20摄氏度，最适宜的水温为10～15摄氏度，水温低于3摄氏度或高于20摄氏度，基本停止生长，这样就形成夏眠和冬眠的潜伏期。

每当夏季来临，海水的温度一天天升高，海参就爬到深水里伏在岩礁缝隙中或石头的附近，不吃也不动，开始"夏眠"，它一直睡到仲秋季节，才开始活动，这一觉足足睡上三个多月！秋高气爽，水温渐凉，海参便爬到浅海中，边爬边觅食，海底含有丰富的有机物和小虫的泥沙，吞噬下去，夹在泥沙中的小虫和有机物被消化吸收，消化不了的泥沙被排出体外。然而这些粪便却给潜水员捕捉海参提供了线索。

每当入冬水温下降了3摄氏度时，即进行12月至来年3月的冬眠，这一觉又睡了三个多月，这样就

后　记

《中华百草御膳》一书终于完稿了，看着这多年心血的结晶，怅然之情，难以言状。回首二十年的烹饪之路，不知是甜，是苦。

在《中华百草御膳》即将出版之即，首先要感谢曾经把我领进烹饪殿堂的启蒙老师们，还要感谢国宝级烹饪大师们的多年无私指导、教诲。他们是：京菜大师金勇泉，粤菜大师康辉，宫廷菜传人董世国，谭家菜第三代传人陈玉亮、鲁菜大师孙仲才、时广南，清真菜大师马景海，素菜大师林月生，冷菜大师董玉昆等，许多烹饪前辈，在我的烹饪成长之路中凝结着他们的经验和智慧。更要感谢王涤寰老师的热情帮助，特别是他的精彩摄影，使菜肴更加生辉。

在本书的制作过程中我的同事们更是倾力相助，书中也包含着他们的智慧和劳动。他们是：药剂师孙磊、烹调师施玉海、孔德旭、宋伟、张宝、杨军山、张刚及狄杰、闫志松、张斌、赵立文……。

中国烹饪渊源几千年，发展到今天，健康饮食已成为不可逆转的时尚。但愿这本以美味为基础，以推动健康饮食为目的的拙作，能起到抛砖引玉的作用，使从事烹饪工作的专业人士和全社会的人们，注重饮食养生，以强健我们的民族，乃至促进全人类的健康。

由于水平有限，在编纂过程中定有许多欠妥之处，敬请老师、同行们提出意见。

多谢！

焦明耀
2001 年 10 月 1 日于北京

Postscript

《The Chinese Herb-medicine Imperial Cuisine of Nourishing Life》 has been finished finally. It is hard to express my feeling when I see the fruit of painstaking labor of many years. To review the cooking route of twenty years that I don't know whether it is sweet or bitter.

At this time of publishing of 《The Chinese Herb-medicine Imperial Cuisine of Nourishing Life》, I'll thank the teachers who introduced me to the field of cooking. I'll also thank the national treasure class cooks for their disinterested guide and teaching. They are great master of Jing dish, Jin Yongliang; great master of Yue dish, Kang Hui, the person who inherits and passes on the palace dish of learning, Dong Shiguo; the third generation who inherits and passes on Tanjia dish of learning, Chen Yuliang; great master of Lu dish, Sun Zhongcai and Shi Guangnan; great master of Qingzhen dish, Ma Jinghai; great master of vegetable dish, Lin Yuesheng, great master of cold dish, Dong Yukun. My growing road of cooking is embodied these great masters' experience and intelligence. Especially, I'll thank the teacher, Wang Dihuan's warm-hearted help. His wonderful photographs make the dishes more splendid.

During the writing, my associates tried their best to help me and this book also contains their intelligence and labor. They are the druggist, Sun Lei; the cooks, Shi Yuhai, Kong Dexu, Song Wei, Zhangbao, Yang Junshan, Zhang Gang, Di Jie, Yan Zhisong, Zhang Bin and Zhao Wenli, etc.

The cooking of China has several thousand year's history. Today, the fashion of healthcare diet can not be reversed. I hope this book on the bases of dainty and on the purpose of promoting the healthcare diet can cause the effect of casting in brick to attect jade to make the specialists dealing with the cook and the people in the society pay more attention to nourishing diet to enhance the health of our nation and promote the people's health.

There must be some deficiencies in the book due to my limited level. so I sincerely hope that the teachers and associates can give your opinions.

Thanks a lot!

Jiao Mingyao
October1, 2001 in Beijing